Astrologers

& Laypersons

Guide

To Medicine

Learn how to do your own formulas with the simple
form of
correlation and with the help & Faith of the Magi –
initially Astrologer Priests & 3 Wise Men

By Di Smith

Future Books:
Astrology and Murder
Astrology and Politics (Autobiography)

*

*

Contents

Authors Natal Chart

Chart 1

DIANE
Natal Chart (624)

2:15 am AEST -10:00
Sydney, NSW
33'S52' 151'E13'
Geocentric
Tropical
Placidus
True Node

ii

Australia's Constitution for NSW Natal & Progressed Chart Given as Reference to- - ABS - Highest Causes of Death

Chart 2

Inner Wheel
Aust'n C'wealth 1-1-1901
Natal Chart (772)
1 Jan 1901
11:00 am AEST -10:00
Sydney, NSW
33°S52' 151°E13'
Geocentric
Tropical
Placidus
True Node

Outer Wheel
Natal Chart (773)
31 Dec 2014
6:14 pm AEST -10:00
Sydney, NSW
33°S52' 151°E13'
Geocentric
Tropical
Placidus
True Node

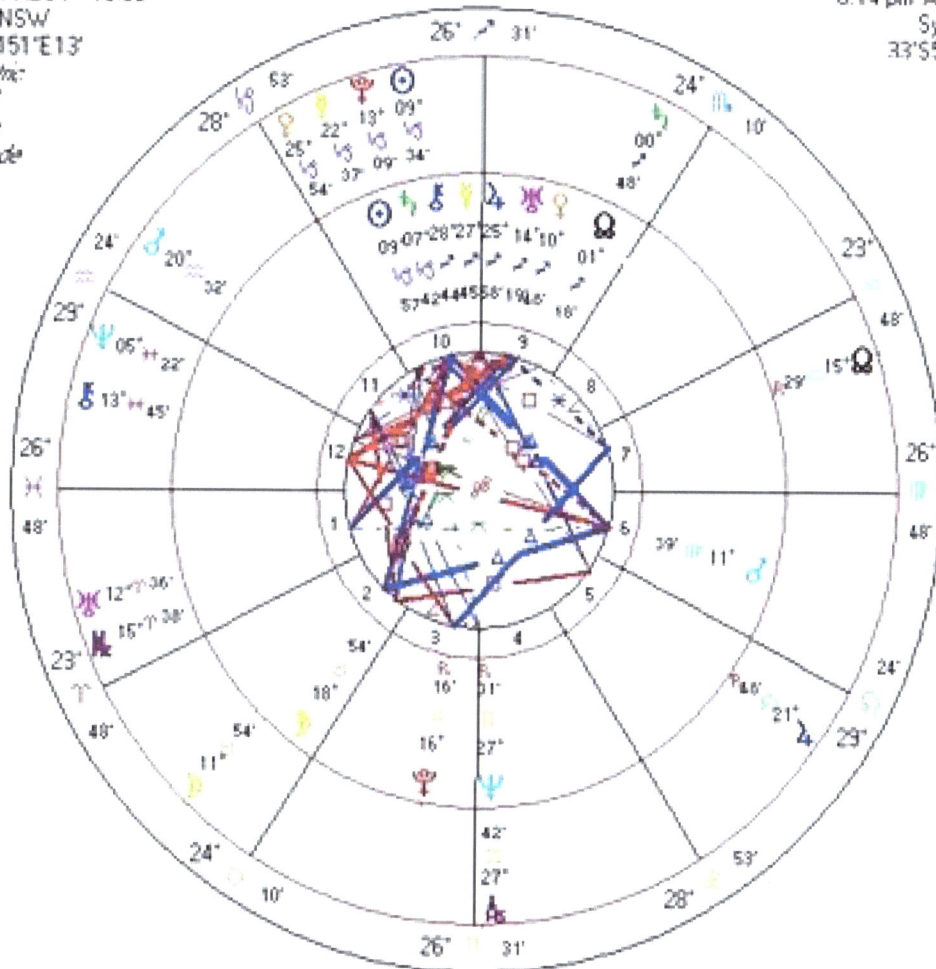

AUSTRALIA'S NATAL & PROGRESSED FLOW CHART FOR 2014WHICH ILLUSTRATES THE FLOW OF PLANETS ONTO ANOTHER

Australia's Natal and Progressed Flow Chart for 2014

Degree '	Planet	Hse		
01 Sag 18	Nth Node	9th	⊼	NN - Venus
02 Tau 33	Venus	2nd		
04 Tau 08	Sun	2nd		
05 Cap 23	Chiron	10th		
07 Cap 42	Saturn	10th		
09 Cap 57	Sun	10th		
10 Sag 48	Venus	9th	□	Venus - Mars
11 Vir 39	Mars	6th	□	Mars - Uranus
13 Cap 00	Jupiter	10th	□	Jupiter - Mercury
14 Sag 26R	Uranus	9th	☍	Uranus - Pluto
14 Ari 30	Mercury	1st	□	Mercury - Saturn
16 Gem 13	Pluto	3rd	⊼	Pluto - Saturn
16 Cap 23	Saturn	10th		
16 Sag 26R	Uranus	9th	⊼	Uranus - Moon
18 Tau 54	Moon	2nd	□	Moon - Mars
25 Leo 27	Mars	5th		
25 Sag 58	Jupiter	9th	☍	Jupiter – Neptune
27 Gem 04	Neptune	4th	☍	Neptune - Mercury
27 Sag 45	Mercury	10th		

United States Declaration of Independence Natal and Progressed Chart for 2 July 1776 – 4 July 2016

Chart 3

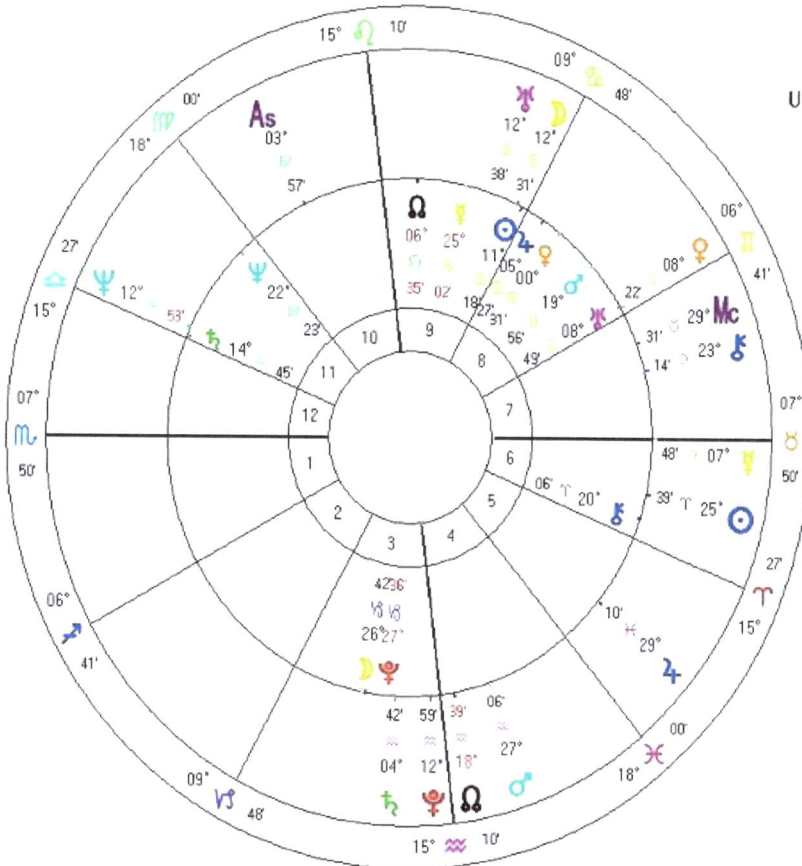

Inner Wheel

U.S. Declaratiom
of Independence

Natal Chart (13)
2 Jul 1776 NS
2:25 pm LMT +5:00:39
Philadelphia
39°N57'08" 075°W09'51"
Geocentric
Tropical
Placidus
True Node

Outer Wheel

U.S. Declaration

of Independence
US prog – Independence
Pennsylvania

Tert.Prog. SA in Long [141]
4 Jul 2016
2:25 pm LMT +5:00:39
Philadelphia
39°N57'08" 075°W09'51"
Geocentric
Tropical
Placidus
True Node

SYMBOL OF CONSTELLATIONS

v

Ram - Male Sheep

 Aries

 Scales + Male/Female

 Libra

 Bull

 Taurus

 Water Scorpion

 Scorpio

 Twins - Two Females

 Gemini

 Centaur Horse Man

 Sagittarius

 Crab

 Cancer

 Goat

 Capricorn

 Lion

 Leo

 Water Bearer

 Aquarius

 Virgin

 Virgo

 Fish

 Pisces

SYMBOL OF PLANETS

Symbols of Planets

Symbol	Name	Abbr	Symbol	Name	Abbr
☽	Moon	Mon	♄	Saturn	Sn
⊕	Earth	Ear	♅ , ♅	Uranus	Ura
☉	Sun	Sun	♆	Neptune	Nep
↓	Vulcan	Vul	♇ , ♇	Pluto	Plu
☿	Mercury	Mer	☊	North Node	Nod
♀	Venus	Ven	☋	South Node	Sno
♂	Mars	Mar	⚷	Chiron	Chi
♃	Jupiter	Jup			

List of Characteristics of Constellations from Aries to Virgo

♈ ♂ 1st	♉ ♀ 2nd	♊ ☿ 3rd	♋ ☽ 4th	♌ ☉ 5th	♍ ☿ 6th
I am	I have	I Think	I Feel	I Will	I Analyse/ I Serve
Active	Artistic	Air	Babies	Bright/	Analyse
Active	Agriculture	Arms	Calcium	Shining	Colon
Setting	Beauty	Brains	Crab	Confident	Correctional
Courage	Earth	Breath	Children	Entertainer	Critical of
Direct	Farm	Communi-	Emotional	Entertainment	Oneself
Fire/Fiery	Land	cation	Emotions	Fire	Digestive
Head	Homie	Lungs	Family	Heart	System
Impulsive	Jealous	Mimics	Homeliness	Humorous	Earth
Individual	Material	Monkey	Homemade	Husband	Health
Action	Objects	Neighbours	Lakes	King/	Hospitals
Initiative	Neck	/hood	Lime	Queen	Judge
Muscles	Land	Nervous	Mammary	Lazy	Judg-
Own-self	Own	Nervous	Glands	Magnesium	mental
Oneness	Money	System	Memories	Proud	Large -
Penis	Possessive	Paper-	Moody	Regal	Intestines
Potassium	Practical	Work	Mother	Royal	Menial
Quick	Possess-	Ribs	Mud	Self -	Work
Sex	Ions	Siblings -	Past	Control	Nagger
Scars	Same	Brothers	Rivers	Sensitive	Practical
Sheep	sex	/Sisters	Sensitive	Solar	Pure
Work place	groups	Theft	Subconscious	Plexus	Snakes
using sharp	Sensual	Transport	Stomach	Son	Virginal
instruments	Stubborn	Twins	Tenacious	Stubborn	Work
Wounds	Throat	Versatile/	Water	Suns	Work
made	Thyroid	Versatility	Womb	Rays	Place
By sharp				Teenagers	
instruments				Warm Hearted	

List of Characteristics of Constellations from Libra - Pisces

♎/♀ 7th	♏/♇ 8th	♐/♃ 9th	♑/♄ 10th	♒/♅ 11th	♓/♆ 12th
I Balance	I Create	I Perceive	I Use	I Know	I Believe
Air	Bowel	Archer	Ambitious	Airplanes	Alcohol
Arts	Brave	Exaggeration	Business	Air	Cold
Balance	Cruelty	Expansive	Bones	Ankles	Confused
Beauty	Envy	Fire	Carbon	Circulation	Drugs
Borderline	Funerals	Foreignors	Contracts	Fixed	Fear
Borders	Graves	Freedom	Control	Electrical	Feet
Contracts	Jealousy	Gestures	Cold	Eruptions	Film
Cooperative	Masses	Hair	Dominant	Freedom	Fish
Courts	Others -	Hips	Earth	Gambler	Ghosts
Diplomat	Money	Hopeful	Efficient	Groups	Guilt
Friends	Possessive	Impatient	Goal -	Humanitarian	Hotels
Helpful	Priest	Laws	orientated	Intellectual	Inferiority
Indecisive	Priestly	Legal	Goats	Open Minded	Instincts
Kidneys	Pope	Liver	Honors	Progressive	Institutes
Lawyer	Rape	Outdoors	Knees	Radiation	Lakes
Marriage	Real Estate	Outgoing	Marrow	Risk Taker	Losing thngs
Mediator	Reproductive -	Philosophers	Objective	Salt	Lymph -
Music	Organ	Philosophy	Orderly	Shin	Glands
Ovaries	Regeneration	Politics -	Orders	Stubbom	Missing
Partnership	Reserve	from	Professional	Sudden	Pictures
Peacemaker	Resourceful	Overseas	Reliable	TV	Photographer
Pleasure	Water	Punter	Ribs	Uranium	Sleep
Police Officer	Sarcasm	Religion	Self Centred	Uncompromis-	Spiritual
Refinement	Scorpion - Water	Silica	Serious	ing	Sponge
Relationships	Spite	Sports	Solitary	Unpredictable	Subconscious
Scales	Stubborn	Sports Arena	Structure		Surrender
Soda	Sulfur	Theatrics	Vertebrae	Volcano	Swimming
Sweetness	Transformation	Thighs		Water -	Tired
Urinary -	True Friend	Travel		carrier	Unconscious
Track	Truth	Undiplomastic		Wilderness	Water
		University		Windy	

Chapter 1 - Australia's & Ors Health Aspects for Sceptics

For people who wish to be healers it will take a leap of faith to make formulas using my correlations. I've found I have to combine colours and you will have to learn the colours. From the colours of Constellations/Planets & Houses you need to find the foods under those signs which combine and have the same colours of the Constellation/Planet or House. This may sound confusing but as you read individual sections hopefully it will all come together.

Sceptics often need proof and I can't say I haven't been a sceptic myself, but, what I'm about to share with you is my greatest secret and the simplest of formulas, and I'd like to be given the credit for finding them after they had be written in black and white for thousands of years without us even realizing it.

Would you believe the Zodiac symbols of Constellations give us our first clue.

1. Aries symbol is the Male Sheep, a Ram - it rules the head and muscles; if you have temperature or a cut, problems with muscles, look there for a curer.
2. Taurus symbol is the Bull, the Male Cow – it rules the neck and thyroid and growth hormones. The oil of a cooked piece of meat does wonders for sore throats.
3. Gemini symbol is the twins. It has to do with humans – so naturally I've looked at alternatives. It rules lungs/Respiratory System/brain and arms. I found the Comfrey flowers were called a 'hand' and will help with the brain.
4. Cancer symbol is the Crab – it rules the stomach/breasts and mammary glands and on the psychological level memories & helps to control worry.
5. Leo symbol is the Lion and China already has it medically recorded as being honored – in using colour association Leo rules the Sun it's colour is orange and I've experimented with Oranges and found if you squeeze one in hot water it immediately removes symptoms of heart problems. There are various ways of using any of them.

From what I've given you, you can work the rest out for yourself.

Now I'm moving onto Australia's Health issues, the following is from the ABS for various years, it's a record of what Doctors have recorded as leading diseases to sudden death.

We don't often realize that the area we live can be a major problem to our health. I felt if I can show you how a countries planets show illness it will help you to understand the theory behind the formulas.

LEADING CAUSES OF DEATH – Australia – Selected years – 2005, 2009, 2014

Cause of death	2005	Rank	2009	Rank	2014	Rank
Ischaemic heart diseases	20 570	1	22 587	1	20 173	1
Dementia, incl. Alzheimers	4 653	5	8 280	3	11 965	2
Cerebrovascular diseases	11 513	2	11 216	2	10 765	3
Trachea, bronchus & lung cancer	7 399	3	7 786	4	8 251	4
Chronic lower respiratory diseases	5 428	4	5 984	5	7 810	5
Diabetes	3 529	8	4 176	6	4 348	6
Blood & Lymph cancer (including Leukaemia)	3 614	7	3 811	8	4 275	7
Colon, sigmoid, rectum & anus cancer	4 171	6	4 068	7	4 169	8

The above is the statistics from the ABS on leading causes of death in Australia. As can be seen it is Ischaemic Heart Disease which includes angina, blocked arteries of the heart and heart attacks. These 3 illnesses are very different. The death number for 2014 was 20,173, over 10 years, it's been said it's steadily been increasing. This is interesting because planets do move and a lot slower when looking at progressions. Instead of the Sun moving 1 degree/day it moves 1 degree in a year, refer the heading 'PLANETS MOVEMENTS'.
.

I've put into my Astrology program, Solar Fire the time of our first Constitution as 11:00 am, the time based on when New South Wales accepted the Constitution. In the above charts I've not only worked on progressions but also transits for when ABS gave the last statistic in 2014.

Really the population affected by the diseases is a drop in the ocean if you calculate the spread over the States and Territories, per year it has raised to 20,173 we have a population of approximately 25 million, we've lost more people in war. Most countries have a great deal higher population and their illnesses are far greater.

In this section I'd like to show how we can see the illnesses by the different planets/constellations/houses. Death is ruled by Pluto.

When we look at the heart in Astrology we are looking at the Leo ♌ Constellation, Sun the planet, and the 5th house. When thinking of the heart I would think of the constellations which naturally oppose and square being Aquarius/Scorpio & Taurus and notice progressed Mars in Leo/5th house, nothing too drastic with that, but it would mean in most cases the heart would be over heated especially with a trine 60° angle to Jupiter. So now I look to the planets. The planets that affect the heart are Saturn which causes calcification/blockages and Pluto obvious death. I'd also look to planets and degrees that are opposite ♂, square □ and 150 degree angles with the symbol ⚟.

Now let's look to Australia's Chart 2. What I see first is that the Sun ☉ is in Capricorn ♑ where the planet conjuncting it is Saturn ♄ . To emphasis this, it is also the planet which rules Capricorn and in the 10th House wooow, this would mean there's a lot of pressure to work, there would also be a lot of constraint, and progressed Saturn is making a 150° to Pluto. This is shown by the influences of Pluto both in progressed and natal chart, outer and inner wheel of chart 2.

Over 115 years Saturn has progress back to where it had been conjunct the Capricorn Sun. It's now at 16° making that 150° angle to Pluto♇ which is also 16°; something that is very important to notice sudden death as it is opposing Pluto is Uranus ♅. This in itself gives an understanding to why Ischaemic disease is the highest death rate in Australia.

Looking at it more in medical terms; Pluto rules the Reproductive System and those hormones associated, whilst Uranus rules our Circulatory System it also sends and electrical pulse through our system and is the water carrier of our body. It's the salts in our body which help the blood to move on along with the Muscular System. These are the areas that would be totally blocked.

Heart patients are probably being restricted salt with Saturn making that 30° aspect to Uranus. But, if we didn't have salt we'd find the nervous system wouldn't work and there probably be problems with breathing, as well, the immune system would shut down as it's related to the white blood cells, and of course problems with the heart, the heart needs a small amount of salt to keep the muscle functioning. This is because the planet Uranus is Aquarius's planet and its natural tissue salt is Nat Mur in simple terms salt, and there is natural opposition to Leo.

Because of the degree and house where Pluto is seen we can also surmise that air, the element of Gemini is being blocked by Pluto, the liver would be working unpredictably and it would have allowed calcification to build up. Uranus is only 3 minutes past Saturn at a 30° angle. Where the affect would be to make the liver work harder. Pluto opposite Sagittarius would stop the air from reaching the liver apart from it working unpredictably.   Because whilst signs are opposite they are dependent on each other to run properly.

The Sun squaring Mercury would show a blockage of air to the heart and with the above would contribute to heart disease.

With all this being said it is relative to a person's/countries chart. But, to me it gives a good indication as to why Australia's no.1 sudden death killer is problems with the heart.

In America Strokes are around the 3rd leading cause of death and it rates around the same for Australia whilst it's not in the above ABS record. When we know what an illness is we can then look to what is causing the problem. For instance, a Stroke is air being blocked to the brain. The brain/air/lungs is ruled by Gemini/Mercury & 3rd house; it is usually caused by a hemorrhage which is caused by leaking of the red blood cells, red blood cells are ruled by Aries/Mars ♂ & 1st house.

In America's chart we see as in Australia's chart Pluto in 3rd house (in a zodiac chart ruled by Gemini) it has an Air Element; In America the constellation Pluto is now in Aquarius also has an Air Element. If you look at America's chart, you'll see prior to Pluto at 12°, Mercury ☿ at 7° in Taurus , 6th house, and these two constellations are squaring each other at a 90° angle. Another aspect to Pluto, the 3rd house with Aquarius over it, is the 150° aspect being made to and from the Sun 11°, progressed Moon 12° 31' and Uranus 12° 38' in Cancer.

This means that Pluto would be making a blockage to air and when air is trying to be pumped to the lungs/brain. In another area regarding the Air Element is whilst it doesn't make a bad aspect to Mercury but its influence will flow onto it is the placing of Uranus in 8th house, and Gemini being its constellation shows again blockage in communications – Gemini and Uranus's Air being blocked by the 8th house ruled by Pluto. In an alternate theory Uranus rules population, Mercury rules neighbourhood and 8th house rules masses. With this theory it does explain how their population has reached 320 million at the start of 2015, Neptune and Saturn making a trine. This is followed with a trine with progressed Neptune to progressed Pluto, soon Neptune will pass Pluto.

The aspects of Pluto is why I'll never consider Pluto as a minor planet, it illustrates where you can find death and with the spiritual side of it remake or rebirth.

There are many other aspects in America's chart but I'm just wanting to focus on Stroke aspects.

Whilst this book is on Health Formula's and how to create them, readers might be enthused to know that I've have taken it another degree, separate to looking at personalities and looking into the future, I have created several environmental formulas. As I didn't have facilities to prove my theories the last formula I requested reviews through the Environment and Scientific Minister Sen. Kerr in 2007-8-9 my formulas were based on Carbons for disabling Uranium. To this date I haven't checked if they've been used.

Most of my initial formulas on the environment I would find patented after requesting reviews, usually 2 years later, by an unknown source. One I still require information on was on eliminating carbon causing Ozone depletion. I asked John Howard, Australian Prime Minister to request NAZA put it on the MIR Satellite a Crystal. I've been told diamonds were found surrounding it when it came down. When requesting a copy, P.M.'s office said they didn't scan letters in the late 90's and my formula would have been forwarded on to the appropriate dept., which they didn't keep particulars of. Would you believe because I was doing investigations into ITSA, I found a lot of unrelated emails/faxes forwarded to them. The blockage for inventions ruled by Uranus is obvious in Australia's chart and communication blockage and pollution/corruption of ideas is obvious with our common and most earthy language with the allowance of f..k, sh.t, in anatomy these areas point to one part of the body which you can find prevalent in Australia's chart; and other profanities, our coarse language is always noticed in American movies. At a time when the country wanted course language to be banned swearing was so imbedded that our laws changed from no swearing to, if it is accepted in the community you're in, it is not illegal.

Chapter 2 - The Medical, Physiology & Anatomy Connection Between The Close Constellations

The importance between the close constellations prior and after have gone quite unnoticed in astrological texts, yet I first came across the importance of this when making formulas and using the 150° angles. I realised it made a figure 8 and in maths the figure 8 stands for infinity. This is not to underrate Square and Oppositions. The 150° angles have a underlining influence, whilst the square and opposition have obvious influence. I also found that the sign prior has an alleviating influence which is why I've written the chart below.

A few years ago I had cause to put the theory in practice for myself to a doctor in the emergency ward who was about to release me after I was admitted with high blood pressure and it had come down. As soon as I got up I realised I wasn't well at all, I couldn't stand. The pain was causing me to have laboured speech where I suddenly found the doctor actually listening to me. I informed him that through astrology the pain in my knees was caused through a problem with oxygen and the heart.

My brain doesn't always tick over to put things into a layperson's term and I was as much amazed, as he was when I came out with it. The information allowed him to do the correct tests to find the problem. I was ecstatic. 1. That the doctor understood what I was saying and 2. finding a diagnosis from the symptoms were almost immediate. Later that day when I was home it was in the Australian news that a scientist in England found a sports person had heart problems, which caused failing knees. Gee I'm almost over it. The amount of times I'm researching something, maybe send it off to a Minister to get government review and proof to my research, to find someone else patents it or claimed recognition for it has been never ending, what's more annoying is the Patents Office is allowing whole area and not a specific area to be patented.

But it's a story of untimeliness. Hopefully this will be timely for someone. Distraction is also another problem, so let's get back to it. ☺

To explain my thoughts in telling the doctor that oxygen and heart were involved in causing my knees to fail, I'll go to the 150° angles in the diagram below. In my case it was the Knees which are Capricorn ♑. The result was that they found I had low oxygen pressure in my arteries. The test is not usually recommended as apparently it's dangerous but I agreed. I needed to know. It was called the Rapid System Text, for myself, I'd say it might be invasive & dangerous if not in a hospital, but you're in the best place if you're going to have heart failure or a stroke. The Dr. punctured me 8x before a registrar helped. It was hard to believe when Dr's said I had to go back to emergency for a check-up they told me it was too invasive. Another reason I look into my own formulas.

Knees & Blockage

♑

150 deg ⇨   ⇦ 150 deg

Gemini Air Ⅱ   ♋   ♌ Fire Leo
Oxygen   Heart

The 150° Angles

In the following I've begun with structuring the constellations by their symbols, food types, cell salts and area of the body they cover and then the second column covers the previous sign that will alleviate the problems of the next. In other chapters I've gone into details of others areas that can cause health problems. So remember it's only when there are planets in these signs are they set off by other influences. Formulas aren't usually made with one ingredient. And, if you ever hear a person say 'I don't like say Pisces because it's opposite my sign of Virgo' please remember that usually in making a formula I always need the opposite or squaring signs ingredient to complete it.

By recognising the below is how I realised the importance of the above.
I've gone through the constellations the first columns going down in order beginning with Aries. The second column is showing the influence of the sign before, Pisces - where the theory is the sign before food can help prevent the next constellation prone to have illness.

Aries - Planet Mars Symbol : Ram/Male Sheep associates : Sheep/Lamb>hogget>mutton. Lamb is high in zinc Abbrev. forms of anatomy: muscles/head, the Brain (Encephalon) Action : Adrenaline & production of Blood. Elements : Fire and Cardinal (Cardinal - active) Medical association: iron is required for good muscle building and esp. for red blood cells a necessary balance is required between white blood cells and red.	Pisces is the sign prior to Aries. To prevent muscle disease: Fish the Symbol of Pisces. Most Fish but the fatter the better Fish have unsaturated fat, different to saturated fats found in butter and those known as saturated fats.
Taurus - Planet Venus Symbol : Buffalo/Bull/Male Cow associates : Cow/Veal-Calves Abbrev. forms of the anatomy: Thyroid/neck Action : Thyroid produces hormone that goes to the pituitary gland in the brain, it's function also regulates fat. Elements : Earth and Fixed (Fixed as if immovable) Medical association: Iodine is required for good Thyroid production and found in food where the iodine will be taken up by the thyroid Planet believed to have	To prevent Thyroid disease: The food product is the Ram the Symbol of Aries Ram refers to the adult male sheep & lamb is reported to have no carbohydrates, a good source of protein, hemme iron and zinc and also rich in all Vit. B's and foilate.. Whilst the meat of cattle has high iron content, they are both red meats, what the thyroid would need is the Ram/sheep meat. (Thyroid Hormone from Wikipedia, the free encyclopedia (Redirected from Thyroid hormones))
Gemini - Planet Mercury Symbol : Twins associates : Human faces showing two sides & areas that have direct access to the brain Abbrev. forms of the anatomy: Lung/brain and arms. Elements : Air and Mutable (Mutable - talkative) Planet believed to have silver and mercuric	To prevent Lung disease: Buffalo the Symbol of Taurus Veal is high in iron potassium. Thyroid hormones are released into the pituitary gland in the brain and T3 and T4 are released into the arms
Cancer - Planet Moon Symbol : The Crab associates : Crayfish Abbrev. forms of the anatomy: Stomach/breast - mammary glands. Action : Acids that break down food from digestive track Elements : Water and Cardinal (Cardinal - active). Abundancy of Oxygen, Iron & Silica	To prevent Stomach disease : The Twins the Symbol of Gemini It is quite likely the Gas Mercury - Mercuric Chloride is the substance found in the lining of the lungs that tells the brain what is good and bad. The Brain then informs the stomach when to purge and when to continue processing the food.
Leo - Planet Sun Symbol : The Lion associates : Tiger/Leopard Abbrev. forms of the anatomy: Heart/Solar plexus Element : Fire and Fixed (Fixed as in immovable)	To prevent Heart disease : The Crab the Symbol of Cancer would be beneficial to heart disease.

Virgo - Planet Mercury Symbol : The Virgin associates : Virginal Abbrev. forms of the anatomy: Intestines Elements : Earth and Mutable (Mutable - talkative)	To prevent Intestinal disease : The Lion is the Symbol of Leo and therefore the meat and even the Heart would stop intestinal problems.
Libra - Planet Venus Symbol : Scales associates : balancing emotions, but can also mean physical anatomical scale, scales on fruit and scale insect - also the metal of a physical scale Abbrev. forms of the anatomy: Kidneys Elements : Air and Cardinal (Cardinal - moveable)	To prevent Kidney disease : The Virgin is the Symbol of Virgo as we are not people eaters another anaylsis is used this can apply to any constellation element. Separate to the symbol but connected to the chemical rulership whilst there are many - the winding long bean are high in the tissue salt
Scorpio - Planet Pluto Symbol : Scorpion associates : Scorpion poison Abbrev. forms of the anatomy: Penis, Vagina, Womb, Bowel, Anus. Elements: Water and Fixed (Fixed as in immovable)	To prevent reproductive organ diseases : The Scale is the Symbol for Libra and given the variety of interpretations the scales on the human body, fruit, fish etc are all possibilities Separate to the symbol but connected to the chemical the Kidney bean or anything in a Kidney shape in the right color.
Sagittarius - Planet Jupiter Symbol : The Archer, on a Horse associates : a Human body on a Horse Abbrev. forms of the anatomy: Liver /Skin /Hips and upper Thigh Elements : Fire and Mutable (Mutable - talkative)	To prevent liver organ disease : The Scorpion is the Symbol of Scorpio the whole animal is used in Chinese medicine it can help the Liver perform its tasks.
Capricorn - Planet Saturn Symbol : The Goat associates : Also known as Buck/Nanny/Billy or Doe/Kid or Mutton in Europe Abbrev. forms of the anatomy: Knees /Bones/ Teeth. Elements : Earth and Cardinal	To prevent bone disease : The Horse is part of the Symbol for Sagittarius, and therefore, the horse and it's Liver can prevent arthritis, rheumatoid arthritis. Osteoarthritis
Aquarius - Planet Uranus Symbol : The Water Carrier associates : Electrical / electrical nerve system /Salt Abbrev. forms of the anatomy: The Circulatory System. and Ankles Elements : Air and Fixed (Fixed as in immovable)	To prevent circulatory disease : The Goat the Symbol of Capricorn and particularly it's knees and cartilage can help the nervous system of the human body and electrodes. I believe it will be found to be high in calcium.

Chapter 3 - PH of Acids and Alkalines; Triplicities and Quadruplicities

With Acids and Alkalines the uneven numbered constellations in the zodiac are alkalines and the even numbered constellations are the acids as shown below:-
Acids & Alkalines

Alkalines:	Aries, Gemini, Leo, Libra, Sagittarius, Aquarius
Fire/Air	Mars, Mercury, Sun, Venus, Jupiter, Aquarius
Acids:	Taurus, Cancer, Virgo, Scorpio, Capricorn, Pisces
Earth/Water	Venus, Moon, Mercury, Pluto, Saturn, Neptune

All the Alkalines are either Fire or Air e.g. Aries - Fire, Gemini - Air, Leo - Fire etc. Acids are put into the triplicities of earth and water respectively. A simple test to find out if something is alkaline or acidic is by using litmus paper it will change from red to blue for alkaline conditions and blue to red for acidic conditions. In numeric form 7 up shows alkaline, and 7 under is acidic.

There are many alkalines and acids of the body which are used by specific organs of the body (which I would say God created, for lack of another description, but there again I believe God created everything) and each do specific things, our body appears to be like a jigsaw puzzle, remarkably everything has a place and required action, what this book is intended to do is to show a link and give an astrological view of anatomy and physiology, which could be added to veterinary studies. I've noticed in Botanists studies colour can contribute to a poison, but in astrology this could be attributed to the area in which the planet is found.

It's been in the botanist's findings have I found plants dispersing gas, which alternately can be formed in the body due to the acids of the body and through oppositions. For me it's exciting to see in the alkaline, it was the first thing that I came across which had the first relationship with something the medical field could understand. In my formulas I often look for an alkaline I can scour to turn into an acid, because in an example I've given further on, an alkaline such as Mars could be in Taurus found under acids.

Our main gas is oxygen which has no ph. So one might presume it has a 7ph I say this because the Sun/Leo is the precursor to it, and Gemini an air sign shows the lungs which it rules causes the oxygenation of the blood all necessary for every part of the body and is caused by photosynthesis made through the earth's atmosphere and the Sun and found mainly by the trees.

As we are taught each sign has a tissue salt we can imagine each of the oxides that would be associated with the Anatomy of the human, in some texts of astrology the Sun rules oxygen because of the photosynthesis it creates, the planet Uranus rules Nitrogen because it is unstable, Hydrogen is ruled by Saturn. In the Zodiac for the Liver, with Jupiter being the ruler we have Silica but if we add one more hydrogen to it, it becomes an acid. The acid grouping for hydrogen is Saturn or Capricorn. For Kidneys they require Natrum Phosphate with Libra and Venus being the ruler, but when Saturn or Capricorn is found affecting Venus ruler of kidneys we could find Cirrhosis a thickening of the kidneys caused by a hydrogen, in astrology hydrogen could create bone growth, nucleus is also ruled by Saturn and the elderly where Nucleic Acid is supposed to be the cause of aging; there are the natural foods to replace this i.e. wheat germ, bran, spinach, asparagus, mushrooms, fish, (esp. sardines, salmon and anchovies), chicken liver, oatmeal and onions. A diet of seafood 7 times a week along with milk and juices.

In the acid family we see constellations and planets that have Earth and Water elements. The stomach ruled by the Moon requires Hydrochloric Acid it requires a degree of acid to breakdown the minerals and foods digested and when there is an upset stomach charcoal is taken. Charcoal is a Calcium but an Earth Calcium, it's a product of potash/burnt wood, whilst Calcium is also an alkaline in Tissue Salts of Cancer, Capricorn and Scorpio, one requires a fluoride, the other a planet food phosphate and the last a Sulphate. Calcium can also be a lime; in an association of words this makes me wonder if the Lime fruit could be used.

From understanding acids and alkalizes we will discover a whole new area giving an understanding to scouring food substances. And, an area the goes more into the terms the medical field understand.

Ionizing is where the chemical reaction takes place for it changes one substance to another. In my studies in Astrology it's caused by planets + specific constellations which have to be counteracted and the best way I've found is by foods making an alkaline food into its acidic form when required.

In the above chart we find a planet and 9th house (ruled by Sagittarius) which are alkaline, and a constellation which is alkaline. Carrots are generally alkaline, when you need an excess of acid the procedure informs you by the elements that there is the requirement for heat, salt water and drying, and therefore the produce needs to be boiled and fire dried. Rice has already been dried and could be ground and added later. Alternately rice flour could be used to thicken it.

Alkaline & Acid Food Types

Alkaline Foods (- ph)
• Vegetables - especially *raw* green leafy vegetables e.g. boiled broccoli, black beans - cooked, green beans - boiled, lima beans - cooked, cucumber peeled, raw cabbage, carrots - boiled, mung bean, , kale boiled, lettuce iceberg, peppers - green sweet and raw, potato - baked with skin, tomato red
• Fresh Herbs and Spices -basil, cilantro, cayenne, ginger, parsley.
• Fruits - apples, avocado, bananas, blueberries fresh, young coconuts, dried dates, grapes fresh kiwi fruit fresh, oranges fresh, strawberries fresh, watermelon,
• Wheat grass.
• Sprouts i.e. alfalfa etc.
• Sour cream

Acid Foods (+ ph)
• Junk and Processed foods.
• Sugar.

- All animal food: - meat – hamburger, turkey, eggs, chicken; fish - catfish baked, lobster, oysters, salmon baked, tuna which is chunky light an canned.
- Grains: (White) wheat, rice pasta flour, bread, garbanzo beans – cooked,
- Some Fruits: - pecans raw, English walnuts raw
- Dairy products: - milk, butter, cheeses i.e. Cheddar, Cottage cheese, Cream cheese – regular, Swiss cheese, plain yoghurt low fat
- Peanuts cashews.

Ref: http://www.thebestofrawfood.com/raw-food-diet-conversion-chart.html
http://www.essense-of-life.com/moreinfo/healthtopics/A-701/foodcharts.htm

The Elements - Triplicities and Quadruplicities

The Triplicities and Quadruplicities give a quick reference to how people will act particularly when there are planets in the constellations. Triplicities give an easy flow, whilst Quadruplicities give a harsh flow.

Triplicities Δ - Trines
The four triplicities and groupings are separated by 120°, the angle primarily refers to the constellation but it could extend to referring to houses and planets as planets rule particular constellations, and houses take on the characteristic of the constellations. The four Triplicities are Fire, Earth, Air and Water.

Often an astrologer will refer to a planet not only a constellation as fixed, active or talkative. In western astrology the Triplicities are Fire, Earth, Air, Water. These groupings cause easy flow and each have a Quadruplicit side to it for when we go around the zodiac we find one is active, the next is fixed and the last is mutable which are the Quadruplicities. The way the constellations flow with Aries ruler of the first house shows if a planet was in that sign it would be active and fiery if there was an affliction by another planet otherwise there could be a warmth and temperate feeling, then when we move to the next easy flow we find Leo, a planet in this house would mean it would be fixed but again if affected the heat of both signs could mean an overheating of the heart, Leo ruler of the heart, this could happen because they mightn't be inclined to act because of the fixed nature, which in fact could be unhealthy, and would probably be more so if it was the Sun in Leo, the next trine is Sagittarius which is mutable/talkative. Planets can make an easy flow to these trines and it is important to understand the temperament of the triplicities. People of the same Triplicities find it easy to either speak, act, be fixed or feel emotional attuned to another person's feelings, water element.

Fire Signs – Aries, Leo, Sagittarius; Mars, Sun, Jupiter, 1st, 5th, 9th house.
Earth Signs – Taurus, Virgo, Capricorn; *Venus, *Mercury, Saturn; 2nd, 6th, 10th house.
Air Signs – Gemini, Libra, Aquarius; *Mercury, *Venus, Uranus; 3rd, 7th, 11th house.
Water Signs – Cancer, Scorpio, Pisces; Moon, Pluto, Neptune; 4th, 8th, 12th house.

Quadruplicities □ Squares
Quadruplicities are groupings of 3 where there are 4 Constellation/Planets and house with same element, separated by 90°, the quadruplicities are Cardinal/Active, Fixed and Mutable, and this

affect goes onto the ruling planet and corresponding house. E.g. Taurus, Leo, Scorpio and Aquarius are all fixed signed when they make their minds up not to do something no one will change their minds, but there are exceptions a father might change a Leo's decision, a group of friends may change an Aquarian person's decision, a fraternity may change a Taurian's mind. The other two are Cardinal and Mutable sign. A group of people with all mutable signs may find themselves talking a lot but not taking too much action; this would be alright in a book club; but, not necessarily good in building a house unless you're the architect, that would be the job of the cardinal signs.

BELOW – THE ELEMENTS FOR CONSTELLATIONS, PLANETS & HOUSES
Cardinal/Active Signs –
> Aries, Cancer, *Libra, Capricorn;
> Mars, Moon, *Venus, Saturn;
> 1st, 4th, 7th, 10th house.

Fixed Signs –
> *Taurus, Leo, Scorpio, Aquarius;
> *Venus, Sun, Pluto, Uranus;
> 2nd, 5th, 8th, 11th house.

Mutable/Talkative Signs –
> *Gemini, *Virgo, Sagittarius, Pisces; *
> **Mercury, Jupiter, Neptune;
> 3rd, 6th, 9th, 12th house.

Astrology is best understood in a simplistic view that by associating words / colour / shape / taste / feel / smell etc. to a particular element /mineral / plant / or animal etc. you'll be surprised how you'll find curers. In other words, each planet rules a colour or colours you can then relate this to the colour of the illness e.g. a person burning with a fever and red hot we'd then be looking for Mars in a chart.

It also has been seen that shape can contribute to cures. This could be explained simply by looking to a walnut and the shape that it gives that resembles the brain and it is believed to help the brain function. . This suggestion may not have been confirmed by the medical profession, as yet, but, in astrology it would be one of the foods used in lung and brain cures, which I'm sure would work if used in the right way and for the right purpose. Something I can confirm is the chestnut 'chest' the impressive word.   I was given a chestnut once from pharmacist when I was deep with congestion, he told me to boil it and inhale, the result was instant, and I think drink the it as tea. The same could be for the walnut boiling and inhaling it, as Gemini is an air sign and rules the lungs, with the prefix being 'wal' and suffix 'nut' if we relate to the shape being round like the head we could summarize that the 'walnut' could help the lining of the head. Please refer photo.

The spear shape of wheat/ barley relates the product of the planet Mars, constellation of Aries it's the warrior with the spear, also Mars relates to sudden cuts and accidents, whilst the product isn't hot, firing it up (as it's a fire sign) could help with pimples in fact I have found the fermenting of things leads to alcohols which can help i.e. whisky, whisky is made from barley, which I've found invaluable with measles; skin aliments are primarily a Jupiter problem and Gin is made from Juniper plant, Sagittarius ruled by Jupiter would be affected by the Moon or Cancer sign, Cancer making that 150 degree orb this would require a product to be fermented; the Moon

12

or Cancer constellation rules the stomach and the action of the stomach is to use hydrochloric acid in the stomach to ferment foods. Cancer sign also has dominance over the mammary glands that produce milk. A common cure for upset stomach is Yakult a fermented milk. If you can see a relationship I used to think to myself and the product is used regularly and it hasn't killed anyone then it's worth a try; with using whiskey on the head for measles not only did it relieve the itching, it brought down the fever.

WHAT YOU SEE COULD BE A CURE?

In the association with words and plants or other products, I have found the Latin/Old Roman and Greek often have meaning behind part of the word with its many variances or other cultures, to the part of the anatomy and tell you which plant will help. Relationship can be found in Botanical names, not necessarily in the full name but by separating it into syllables. I believe, what is generally known through the great tombs of Egypt is that the Pharaohs had a belief structure in astrology and the heavens, which gave us our first hieroglyphics.

13

Chapter 4 - Climate

Climate can affect the health, and we don't often think of it being an alkaline or an acid, and yet perspiration is either an alkaline or an acid and sometimes neutral. Climate can change in one day not necessarily by weather but by the environment that we move to i.e. an air-conditioned building.

In saying that a Climate can be understood by planets, it would probably be affected the most by the moon, and planets that are in your chart combined with others. The moon is very sensitive and rules the emotions and as mentioned the stomach, which can be related to the physical body as below we can also see changes in the atmosphere of countries, personally it is not my field but I will try and explain it:-

Sun is warm to hot and fixed. If there is an affliction it could indicate a person with a high temperature.

Mercury is cold, talkative and an air sign in Gemini but, an earth sign when seen in Virgo, which rules the intestinal area. Environmentally it could indicate a wind that is noisy blowing the leaves through the trees, in health it would indicate extreme barking cough and problems with air.

Venus is dry and fixed or moveable (fixed means will not move until some favorable or unfavorable aspect occurs, Venus is so far the ruler of both Taurus and Venus which is why I've stated 'fixed' and 'moveable') it would indicate an atmosphere that won't move.

Mars is hot and moveable - If a country is in a heat wave we could expect a number of fire signs in a fire constellation. The fire signs are under Quick Reference to Elements.

Moon is warm and moveable. - This would indicate a warm humid atmosphere. It is the fastest planet/satellite of earths that affects it most personally. Within 2 ½ days it would make several aspects to Uranus which is the most unpredictable planet.

Saturn is humid and moveable, and would indicate a cold humid atmosphere, in health it would mean someone who feels clammy.

Jupiter is windy, hot and talkative, with wind there would be the underlying factor of Uranus. Jupiter rules beaches, the wind would bring a relief to the hot weather. And, to explain talkative, the thrashing of the ocean on the beach is heard from the sea waters.

Above are the closest planets to the Sun. But along with temperature some planets have an atmosphere full of gases and the combination of these planets gases can help to alleviate an illness. Instead of dissecting the elements such as seen in the periodic table the planets outline the gases they contain this was given initially by its colour or mixture of colours with primitive or not so primitive telescopes that Astrologers/Astronomers put down to the earth's substances they knew gave a particular colour.

How the illness is formed is through a combination of squares, oppositions and other aspects of planets that can be seen by the degree which are near each other, which one could take quick reference using NASA's Scientist Ephemeris showing planets and their degrees. Planets don't usually move much. Calculations are usually required when the different planets degrees are virtually the same. These planets then oppose or square planets that are conjunct (conjunct – at the same degree). These are obvious illnesses but it is the sesquares and quincunx's that complicate any illness, these are 30 degrees and 150 degree aspects respectively. It is important to remember when making a formula the degree and minute shows us which is prepared first and other planets foods are added if close, within 5 degrees.

The outer planets do play an important part in weather.

Uranus is unpredictable it is air sign so we'd expect winds. It is a fixed sign and how this works could mean that the change that takes place could be at the same time. Like the news stating the temperature will change at a certain time from an easterly. This then could be activated by the Moon being a cardinal/active sign.

Neptune is a water sign and I'm not sure if it has a temperature as such, if you think of a ship in the ocean, where sailors can be on their ship for days on end without a breeze. It takes me back to believing it has to be activated by cardinal sign.

The last is Pluto again this is a water sign. Astronomers have downgraded it to a minor planet. And, there is no proof of Chiron having any real influence except astrologer's stating it is a healer, there is some talk as to whether the Sun goes through its constellation which is believed to be Centaurus, and there talk of a clashing of constellations with Scorpio, in a millions years' time… Pluto is another fixed signed and it stands for disaster at its worst, but, what affect humans is not something that is necessarily detrimental to the earth unless a square or opposition to the Sun. Therefore, if Uranus is making an aspect to Pluto in the 10th house we could see unpredictable volcanos causing the earth to renew itself, or the breaking up of the North and South poles because of Pluto being in Capricorn.

What is said about the outer planets is that they have a characteristic, which happens and affects a generation as they move gigantic things when involved, and, their length of time in a constellation can be considerable e.g. Pluto take 13-32 years to go through one constellation.

Chapter 5 - The Influences of Constellations as Compared to the Planet and House

Below is how I've found to analyze a chart, it's the basics, whilst Arabic astrologers begin their charts with Pisces on the first house, I put Aries on the 1st house, as Western astrologers do and have found no problems in finding formulas, but, Western Astrologers mainly analyze personal planets and how they affect constellations and houses.

The below is how I view things both personal and emotional when trying to find a formula. Illness is not necessarily one thing and if you find there is turmoil in one of the groupings you can look to the inner organ to be upset.

PLANETS MOVEMENTS

The planets movements show how turmoil's can move on, as the inner planets move a lot faster than the exterior.

The planets length of time it takes to circle the Sun are shown below. I've included the Sun but it is really as it's seen from Earth. And, the Moon is actually circling the Earth.

Sun – 25.38 days
Moon – 27.321 days through all the constellations from earth

Below shows the time all other planets take to go around the Sun and through the 12 Constellations an ephemeris is required to see in which constellation they are in and the varying length of time they're in it.

Mercury – 88 days, Mercury is only ever 28 degrees away from the Sun and can spend only 4 days in one sign.
Venus – 245 days through all constellations
Earth – 365.24 days through all constellations, it's the Earths view of the Sun that we see Sun move through the Constellation, it'*s the degree that we judge our Zodiac sign or Sun sign, which most people are interested in.
Mars – 687 days
Jupiter – 11.86 years, spends approximately 1 year in each sign
Saturn – 29 ½ years = 10,759 earth days spends approximately 2 ½ year in each sign.
Uranus – 84 earth years
Neptune – 164.79 years
Pluto - 284 days can spend 13-32 years in a sign.
The Chart below shows Constellation/House/Planet and the Triplicities and Quadruplicities that change them.

Constellation	House - Take from TOB	Planet	Quadruplicity	Triplicity
Aries	1st house	Mars	Cardinal-Active	Fire
Taurus	2nd house	Venus (this is sweet earth)	Fixed	Earth
Gemini	3rd house	Mercury (as in air)	Mutable Talkative	Air
Cancer	4th house	Moon	Cardinal - Active	Water
Leo	5th house	Sun	Fixed	Fire
Virgo	6th house	Mercury (as in earth)	Mutable - Talkative	Earth
Libra	7th house	Venus (this is sweet air)	Cardinal - Active	Air
Scorpio	8th house	Pluto	Fixed	Water
Sagittarius	9th house	Jupiter	Mutable - Talkative	Fire
Capricorn	10th house	Saturn	Cardinal - Active	Earth
Aquarius	11th house	Uranus	Fixed	Air
Pisces	12th house	Neptune	Mutable - Talkative	Water

By following this you'll be able to relate to the planet and house, and constellation ALSO known as the sign. The Constellation is the area in the anatomy; the Planet is the influence or what's being brought into the area and the house shows the area of the body that is being affected.

The Quadruplicities and Triplicities are elements which are extremely important in analyzing for instance Aquarius is fixed and so is a trunk of a tree, the croton tree is specific to Aquarius the *Croton tiglium tree* is medical use is for healing lesions; severe constipation as a purgative, it is used in wind breaks ; In the Amazon the red latex from the species *Croton lechleri*, known as Sangre de Drago (Dragon's blood), is used as a "liquid bandage". Another interesting point is that it's been found to be a source of the organic compound *phorbol and its tumor promoting esters*, analyzing 150 degree angle Aquarius is an underlying problem for Cancerians https://en.wikipedia.org/wiki/Croton_(plant) I should stress a person who's born the zodiac sign of Cancer is not necessarily going to die of Cancer; health problems are determined by ill placed planetary aspects.

By understanding the elements actions e.g. if Mars was in the 2nd house ruled by Taurus, the person is likely to bring a warm aspect to the area, would be active in brotherhoods, the place is likely to be where there's male or female bonding, you'd automatically be brought to Mars – warmth or hot and active, Taurus is bonding or same sexes. In western astrology the philosophy begins with Aries once you understand their character you will then see that the three areas use different parts of the characteristic to operate.

Another example is to put Cancer on the Ascendant, which is the first house a person with this aspect would show themselves as being caring and creative in any area there in, they might work hard at keeping the place clean, but using the term 'work' would bring in a Saturn influence, but, it has a natural active nature, I should add in a progress chart the houses will change, the planets move…the following is an explanation to this theory…

Aries- 1st House - Mars

The **constellation Aries** is direct as if they know what they're doing, they're an active sign (active meaning cardinal, and, fiery meaning instantaneous) it has a natural warmth coming due to its fiery element; it gives the want for movement, it's pointed in shape. Its keyword is 'I' The Arian nature gives Taurians the reason for doing what they do. Aries rules the part of the anatomy which is muscles throughout the body and those of the skull and muscle surrounding it. External – the Head.

The **1st house** rules the environment it would be hot, a person's likely to be living in an arid area, may have a pointed roof, possibly red brick, or geographically maybe where wheat is grown or even thistles. In medical terms their head could be hot or whole body. It's the Planets and Constellations that will change it.

The **Planet Mars** shows the influence in the area it is found, Mars is hot, active, i.e. if the planet is afflicted - temperature would go up and down and up again, if afflicted – inflamed and red

Taurus - 2ND House - Venus
(Venus the Earth element as opposed to Libra)

The **constellation Taurus** is fixed and persevering, and earth sign, being fixed means immovable, so when they decide to stop doing something they will not change their minds unless they decide to. Yet their influenced by their male or female counterpart. It rules money, food, possessions, conservative ideas, their conservative ideas are what generally is accepted by those they grow up with. It is also a sign of brotherhood of the same sexes e.g. Freemasons or Country Woman's Association (CWA). They have the ability to continue the Arian dream. Keyword 'I have'. What they do in today's society leads to Gemini. part of the anatomy is the Thyroid/Thymus and the growth hormone, the pituitary gland, this also regulates blood pressure and stress. External- the Neck/ Throat

The **2nd House** rules the environment, the area would be the throat and pituitary gland

The **Planet Venus** is to influence the constellation it's in by the influences of the constellation it rules, medically it could cause the constellation to be sweet, with sugar. As it rules the throat if Venus was in Taurus it would mean a very nice voice.

As an e.g. Mars in Capricorn 2nd house, there would be a lot of action, heat and constraint happening in the thyroid and pituitary gland. Both Mars and Capricorn are active their functions are opposite each other, their colours are red, black and pink.

Gemini - 3rd House - Mercury

(Mercury the Air Element as opposed to Virgo)

The **Constellation Gemini's** part of the anatomy is the lungs, brain which rules the breathing process which leads us to the action to push through air and here we can also see the muscles action of the earlier sign in the lung which would be the testosterone, which would not even be thought of. Externally - the arms.

19

The Planet Mercury is talkative and versatile in their thoughts with an air element. The planet Mercury causes a person to talk on varying aspects of constellation it's in and the aspects affecting it. Talkative meaning mutable and versatile from being an air sign, it will be talkative in whatever area you find Gemini/Mercury, planet and 3rd house. It rules siblings, the neighbourhood, early schooling, transport and communicates/communication, correspondence. Keywords 'I have an idea'. It's anatomy is the Brain and Shoulder and Arms E.g. Mercury in Capricorn prone to talk about work.. It brings air/oxygen & earth into the equation,

The **3ʳᵈ House** the environment as known by Gemini, of course its physical area would be the lung or brain. If afflicted, you'd notice problems with breathing, speech and with arranging thoughts, but the area these things would be noticed, in the neighbourhood, with brothers and sisters, in educational areas, possibly using different types of transport. It could even be stressful writing maybe to governments or court hearings.

An example would be, if we saw Mercury in Scorpio in 3ʳᵈ house, it means that air would be affecting the sexual hormone as it's negatively placed, which could be causing problems with communication - 3ʳᵈ house pointing us to the lungs and brain; two air elements 3ʳᵈ house and Mercury means excessive air maybe appearing as hyperventilating. Mercury in Scorpio could also cause a person to talk during sex. Or in a medical sense causing too much wind with too much air; it probably wouldn't be too good for a spy.

Cancer - 4ᵗʰ house - Moon

The Cancer Constellation is sensitive in their actions, and is an active sign being cardinal, and watery. It rules family, babies and children and the home and needless to say 'tears'. It also rules the emotions/ memories and habits. Keyword 'I care' It's anatomy is the Breast/Mammary Glands and Stomach its role is to produce hydrochloric acid that breaks down foods.

The Moon brings with it feeling. Its physical aspect is water, it can worry about things and its sensitivity causes it to withdraw if challenged, this would be seen in the area of the constellation. As with it counterpart the Moon would bring into the area hydrochloric acid and only would affect those areas which are square and opposite and making 150-degree angle.

The **4ᵗʰ House** position as with other houses are only affected if there is a planet in them, or those that contradicts the house or constellation it's in. Where there is an upset you'd find it would be noticed in the home or with family, and around babies. A mild case would be heartburn.

Leo - 5ᵗʰ House - Sun

Leo Constellation is fixed and fiery, proud and sensitive (a characteristic formed from Cancer), it rules teenagers, entertainment, the soul/the self, it's royal and can indicate Royalty. Keyword 'I am', without being sensitive it wouldn't notice the admiration of others to feel proud and can lead to being vain, as with myself not wishing to go out without my hair done. People may think this is just a Leo sign, I'd like to explain the Sun which rules Leo can be in any of the 12 signs and where ever, that is, is where a person feels Proud, even if they don't know it. it's known as the zodiac sign, but more of that under Sun. Its anatomy is Chest and the Heart Organ, the atrium, the ventricles and the pulmonary areas, And there is a close relationship with the opposite sign which rules circulatory system. Itself gives out warmth which often goes unnoticed, it's also one of romance, where ever the constellation is in your chart, there's also an interest in helping youth groups, this is mainly seen if there are planets in and making an aspect to it.

The Sun takes approx. 30 days to go through constellations which is the dominant factor in the zodiac. It's royal, it shows pride, it's influence is seen by individual zodiacs more than any other planets. The heart would be affected if afflicted by 150 degree angles by other planets and constellations, but naturally with squares and oppositions.

The 5th **House** is the area of entertainment and will depict where youth groups meet. It will be noticed if planets are in it and afflicted by other planets. It's also the house of romance. E.g. if the Planet Pluto is in Taurus in the 5th house; Pluto would make the person appear quiet yet powerful, when in the 5th house it would be noticed in groups the opposite sign Aquarius rules; they would be the one to stand out and do things by themselves, Pluto, Taurus in 5th house could mean too much acidity in the heart and hormonal test might show it's being absorbed by the heart where they could be overeating causing cholesterol problems. If there are no other planets and constellations affecting it there might be no problems other, then weight.

Virgo - 6th House - Mercury

(Mercury the earth element, as opposed to Mercury created for inhaling .02mg)

The Virgo Constellation is talkative and prudent in the earth sign, it is also practical and can be critical of themselves and others, looking for perfection, it indicates a way and area in which one works. Keyword 'I can' It is virginal and bring about the attitude of no sex in the work are, it's an area and sign where they want to be of service but it also rules computers and working with small things. Its anatomy is the Small and Large Intestines. As the intestinal area is quiet twisting it is interesting to note that snake venom, snake penis, are offered in Chinese Medicine as good for the intestinal region and for intestinal upset.

6th House is where a person will find the type of work they'd be suited to; it is where they want to be of service. It points to the intestinal region if afflicted.

Mercury the ruler of both Virgo or Gemini will only take on the Virgo thoughts if in Virgo constellation. It is strange that the great Astrologer/Astronomers chose this planet for both signs as the Constellations are squaring each other. It will take on the illness of the Planets and those Constellation which affects it.

Libra - 7th House   Venus

The Libra Constellation is active and an air sign it acts in partnership, and shows a caring for their partner and what together they can do. When activated by a planet there would be a love in whatever they do. Keywords 'We can'. A plant that is coupled or shaped like a kidney i.e. a kidney bean or kidney meat are all in helping a healthy kidney. Needless to say it's anatomy rules the Kidneys and associated areas.

The 7th House is one of partnership. In illness it points to the Kidneys and Urinary Track.

The Planet Venus rules both Libra and Taurus. In Libra it rules love of partnership, it's active/cardinal and has an air element, which means it like to talk about the things they love. I have often combined the Taurus and Libra elements to come to a product i.e. sweet meat. Taurus is shown by the buffalo and rules meat, and I'd look for an alkaline product which is sweet to combine it.

Scorpio - 8th House - Pluto

The Scorpio Constellation is fixed and have deep concepts it rules real estate, regeneration, death, the responsibility of other people's money, and sex. It also rules the masses. It has the strongest faith when it decides upon one, possibly to the point of fanaticism. Scorpions will sting themselves under stress. Keyword 'I manage'. It is the poison of the Scorpio that would be useful in male and female reproductive system, or the end part of the bladder, the vagina and where it involves dead tissue. Its anatomy rules the Reproductive System, the Bowel, Bladder and Vagina.

The 8ᵗʰ House shows the groin and the Reproductive System or bowel would be affected if planets or constellation ruling it were afflicted.

Pluto brings with the influence of the lowest degradation and the highest of honors, the wealthiest of the wealthiest, but there again it will depend on what area it's found and the aspects surrounding it. It will add to a Constellation or House Calcium Sulphate; this can deaden or bring to life whatever the problem is but as you'll see in formulas I've created there is a great deal more involved. Pluto is a generational planet which means it will be in a Constellation for at least 13 years and they say as long as 32 years. By which time there are a generation of people born. It had made a spiritual aspect to Neptune for 15 years before I was born and if I'm right for 15 years + more. It totally tires a person out. You can sleep forever and watch life go by.

Sagittarius - 9ᵗʰ House - Jupiter

The Sagittarius Constellation is talkative and fiery it rules philosophy, sport, and higher education, overseas travel, countries and their people. it is hopeful in nature and speaks of ideologies. The Archer draws its Arrow and knows not where it lies (a philosophy is not necessarily practical), but a skilled archer knows where it lies. Its keyword is 'I philosophies'. In terms of illness it relates to heat and spreading as opposed to concentrated small areas, we could use the product of a horse to stop expansion and calm the liver. It also rules sand and silica. Its anatomy rules the Liver, Skin and Hips.

Something I've found interesting is that in early depictions of the symbol of Sagittarius it showed as a Centuarian a man with a horse's body. As such I've utilized that philosophy and have used a horse's manure and blended it with oil. After telling the volunteer client what I was using of which he agreed to, the symptoms he had went away.

The 9ᵗʰ House points to the Liver and Skin, hips/thighs gluttonous with Venus; if philosophies are being constantly challenged which is the external influence it can affect the internal actions of the liver and hips, and can lead to skin problems. The outside facilities of 9ᵗʰ house are universities, the seaside, sports fields, immigration, airports

Jupiter brings with it hope, optimism, the ability to renew one's faith, just as the Liver can renew and regrow itself. It rules the sands left by the oceans waves, clays with their elasticity and glass as a product of sand. It rules religion, law and philosophy

Capricorn - 10ᵗʰ House - Saturn

The Capricorn Constellation is an earth and active sign, seen by it's triplicities and Quadruplicities; it rules pain, blockages, structure, and government it works towards structuring philosophy or ideologies of the previous sign causing it to become and create businesses. The Goat climbs the mountain to the highest peak. 'I work'. It can be humble always with a view in mind. As an earth product and refined we look to such products as oil, being cardinal, the sign would keep working on its environment, it rules coal, a product of coal is oil which is good for the knees and bones. Another form of Capricorn is bricks and cement. Its anatomy rules Knees and Bones.

10ᵗʰ house points to structure, and in the anatomy what supports the structure, but the knees and bones. It's cell salt is Calcium Phosphate and a product of that is potash. It is recommended that we take calcium for the bones, but not all calcium's are good for the bones which should be looked into. If Saturn wasn't in the 10ᵗʰ house it would mean it was likely that there'd be an absence of courts and government structure. If Saturn was in Taurus we'd probably see Goats as a food source, but, in Australia we have the Moon in Taurus where we are beef eaters and because we have an aspect to 10ᵗʰ house it is a commercialized item and transported overseas. Further investigation shows Venus in Sagittarius making an aspect to Saturn in Capricorn

The Planet Saturn brings with it a structured area; what a person would like to work on, it is serious and determined and rules courts and governments; it will bring with it Calcium Phosphate.

Aquarius - 11th House - Uranus

The Aquarius Constellation is fixed and an air sign, planets seen in this constellation show unpredictability or revolutionary ideas, it rules groups, animals, volcanoes, sudden eruptions. The Water Bearer nurtures. Keyword 'We think' We'd be looking for a food that would be unpredictable, such as mushrooms, this would probably help the circulation. It's anatomy rules the Ankles and Circulatory System.

A product in our oceans is created by the Volcanic reaction producing Chloride Ion mixing with Sodium Ion of the rivers, it would also be boiling underground water and mixing with the Chloride Ion, this creation is the tissue salt of Aquarius and Uranus and would be required by the 11th and 5th house. The basic element is Salt aka Sodium Chloride.

11th house rules groups, whatever Constellation is on this house will show what type of group. The 11th house points to the ankles and how a person circulates.

The Planet Uranus, is where a person or even a country will show their unpredictability and ingenious nature.

Pisces - 12th House - Neptune

The Pisces Constellation is talkative and rules the hidden area i.e. sleep, dreams, sleep talking, hypnosis, meditation, what we say without thinking or even realizing we've said it, it rules drugs and alcohol, ghosts, and, the supernatural, fears and phobias, illusions but also the psychic. In the external world institutes, prisons and mental health, mists, and, the knowing of something before it happens something that has no structure or form. The Fish going in different directions but returning to its group, an inheritance from Aquarius, is a possible reaction to being forewarned on a psychic level, predators of fish are often bigger fish. Its anatomy rules the Feet and Lymph System.

12th house points to the feet and lymph system. Whatever planets are in the 12th house will show the action that will take place on a spiritual or subconscious level. Areas it also points to are spiritual churches, Widgey Board aka Ouija boards, Séances. Environmental areas would be rivers, creeks, gullies where mist might form.

Neptune is the planet that rules the ocean along with Pluto whilst it's symbol is the Scorpion which can be found in many areas land and sea, and a new form with every constellation/house and planet. Neptune brings with it a spiritual or confused aspect or both; a person sometimes finds it hard to come to terms with forgetfulness, where they could have been daydreaming or falling asleep. The cell salt is Ferr Phos. And the quantity would depend on the condition of the illness. Personally I have many Neptune Pisces aspects and take 11 with a 100 in a container I can run out fast, where alcohol can be a substitute.

Chapter 6 - Tissue/Cell Salt Combinations

The Cell Salts of the Body and What They Mean

Below is an outline of the properties of the natural chemicals found in the body, which are connected to various constellations, whilst there are number I'm only referring to 10 of them. The properties can be found in any vitamin book 'The Vitamin Bible' published in 1982 describe them as individually depicted below, the graph shows how various combinations are being used for alternate constellation as such Dr. W.H. Schuessler tissue salts combine these to make the 12 combinations applied to the constellations.

In the late 1900's early 2000, Australia took Schuessler tissue salts off the pharmaceutical list and so they are no longer available in Australia but they are available on the Internet. Their explanation for taking them off the pharmaceutical list and actually not put back on to me appeared strange, for they stated they were not being made in the right proportions.

Personally at the time I was using them frequently, but the dosage was highly increased when taking Ferr Phos. At the time I was severely anaemic which I've gone into in later chapter and as such I was taking 11 Ferr Phos tablets; I wouldn't recommend it for other people unless you've been diagnosed as being extremely low in iron. I even went to the extent of drying my own seaweed because I couldn't buy it from health food stores, but these were not the end all to the treatment I took. I was constantly being monitored by Dr's and would often ask if cell salts would help doctors would often respond that there was no medical research that contradicted them or supported them, so I was told I could give them a try.

When the tissue salts were stopped I began to look into the natural foods more for formula's and found it hard to find books that had a good joint analysis as such I've written out the individual properties below.

PROPERTIES OF INDIVIDUAL MINERALS

CALCIUM - Cancer, Scorpio and Capricorn
There is more calcium in the body than any other mineral.
Calcium and iron are the two minerals most deficient in a woman's diet.

IN ADDITION
Maintains strong bones and healthy teeth.
Keeps your heart beating regularly.
Alleviates insomnia.
Helps metabolise your body's iron.
Aid your nervous system, especially in impulse transmission.

DEFICIENCIES
Rickets, hypoglycaemic, osteomalacia, osteoporosis. Growing pains and backaches could be helped with dolomite, chelate calcium or bonemeal.

BEST NATURAL FOODS
Milk, and milk products, all cheeses, soybeans, sardines, salmon, peanuts, walnuts, sunflower seeds, dried beans, green vegetables.

SUPPLEMENTS
Dolomite is a natural form of calcium and magnesium and no vitamin D is needed for assimilation.

ENEMIES
Large quantities of fat oxalic acid (found in chocolate and rhubarb) and phytic acid (found in grains) are capable of preventing proper calcium absorption.

ZODIAC SIGNS
Cancer – Calc Fluor (Calcium Fluoride); Scorpio – Calc Sulph (Calcium Sulphate); Capricorn – Calc Phos (Calcium Phosphate)

CHLORINE – Gemini and Aquarius
Chlorine regulates the blood's alkaline acid balance.
Aids in the cleaning of the body's waste by helping the liver to function.

IN ADDITTION
Aids in digestion
Help keep the body limber.

DEFICIENCES
Loss of hair and teeth.

BEST NATURAL FOODS
Table salt, kelp, olives.

ZODIAC SIGNS
Gemini – Kali Mur (Potassium Chloride); Aquarius – Nat Mur (Sodium Chloride – Salt)

FLUORIDE – Cancer
Fluoride is found in nature in the compound of calcium fluoride. It is sometimes added to water by the government it was believed it would improve teeth and lessen cavities.

BEST NATURAL FOODS
Fluoridated drinking water, cranberry juice, seafood, blue crab canned and gelatine.

TOXICITY
Severe cases of fluorosis cause the enamel to become pitted and very badly stained. More a problem with children when their teeth are developing.

ZODIAC SIGN
Calcium Fluoride - Cancer

IRON - Pisces
Iron is essential and required for life, necessary for the production of haemoglobin, red pigment in muscles.
Iron and calcium are the two major dietary deficiencies of women.
Only about 8 percent of your total iron intake is absorbed and actually enters your bloodstream

IN ADDITION
Aids growth.
Promotes resistance to disease.
Prevents fatigue.
Cure and prevent iron-deficiency anaemia.
Brings back good skin tone.

BEST NATURAL FOODS
Pork liver beef kidney heart and liver, farina, raw clams, dried peaches, red meat, egg yolks, oysters, nuts, beans, asparagus molasses, oatmeal.

ENEMIES
Phosphoproteins in eggs and phytates in unleavened whole wheat reduce iron availability to body.

ZODIAC SIGN
Pisces - Ferr Phos (Phosphate of Iron)

MAGNESIUM - Leo
Magnesium is essential for effective nerve and muscle functioning.
Important for converting blood sugar into energy.
Known as the anti-stress mineral.
Alcoholics are usually deficient.
The human body contains approximately 21 g. of magnesium.

IN ADDITION
Aids in fighting depression.
Promotes a healthier cardiovascular system and helps prevent heart attacks.
Keeps teeth healthier.
Helps prevent calcium deposits, kidney and gallstones.
Brings relief from indigestion.

BEST NATURAL FOODS
Figs, lemons grapefruit yellow corn, almonds, nuts seeds dark-green vegetables, apples.

ENEMIES
Diuretics, alcohol

ZODIAC SIGN
Leo – Mag. Phos (Magnesium Phosphate)

PHOSPHORUS – Aries, Leo, Libra, Capricorn and Pisces
Phosphorus is present in every cell of the body. The most of it are in the above signs.
It's involved in virtually all physiological chemical reactions.
It is necessary for normal bone and tooth structure and Important for heart regularity and, essential for kidney functions.
Phosphorus is needed for the transference of nerve impulses.

IN ADDITION
Aids in growth and body repair
Provides energy and vigour by helping in the metabolisation of fats and starches.
Lessen the pain of arthritis.
Promotes healthy gums and teeth.

DEFICIENCIES
Rickets, pyorrhea – disease of the tissue that surrounds and support the teeth.

BEST NATURAL FOODS
Fish, poultry, meat, whole grains, **bonemeal,** eggs, nuts seeds.

ENEMIES
Too much iron, aluminium and magnesium can make phosphorus inactive.

ZODIAC SIGN
Aries – Kali Phos (Potassium Phosphate); Leo – Mag Phos (Magnesium Phosphate); Libra – Nat Phos (Phosphate of Soda); Capricorn – Calc Phos (Calcium Phosphate); Pisces – Ferr Phos (Phosphate of Iron).

POTASSIUM - Aries
Works with sodium to regulate the body's water balance and normalise heart rhythms. (Potassium works inside the cells, sodium works just outside them.)

In addition, it can assist in reducing blood pressure, edema, hypoglycaemia (Low sugar).

BEST NATURAL FOODS

Citrus fruits, watercress, all green leafy vegetables, mint leaves, sunflower seeds, bananas, potatoes.

TOXICITY
25 g. of potassium chloride can cause toxicity.

ENEMIES
Alcohol, coffee, sugar, diuretics

ZODIAC SIGN
Aries – Kali Phos (Potassium Phosphate); Gemini – Kali Mur (Potassium Chloride); Virgo – Kali   Sulph   (Potassium   Sulphate)

SILICA - Sagittarius
Silica strengthens the blood vessels, improves elasticity in the joints. Prevents the body from absorbing aluminium and flushes aluminium from the tissues. Delays the tissues ageing process. Increases mobility. Aids in bone healing. Strengthens hair. Prevents wrinkles. Strengthen nails.

IN ADDITTION
Silica is required in walls of our body i.e. tendons, blood vessels, bones, arteries and separately the connective tissue. Aorta contains silica.

DEFICIENCES
Believed to cause Atherosclerosis.
Lack of elasticity in the skin.

BEST NATURAL FOODS
Oats (grounded), celery, yellow peppers, carrots, onions, unrefined grains, potatoes, cereals and white rice, yeast, beetroot.
The herb horsetail.

ZODIAC SIGN
Sagittarius - Silica

SODIUM – Taurus, Libra and Aquarius
Sodium and potassium are both found together and both found to be essential for normal growth. Sodium aids in keeping calcium and other minerals in the blood soluble.

IN ADDITTION
Sodium can aid in preventing heat prostration or sunstroke, and can help nerves and muscles to function properly.

DEFICIENCES

Impaired carbohydrates digestion, possibly neuralgia.

TOXICITY
Diets high in sodium usually accounts for high blood pressure.

BEST NATURAL FOODS
Salt, shellfish, carrots, beets, artichokes, dried beef, brains, kidney, bacon

ZODIAC SIGN
Taurus – Nat Sulph; Libra – Nat Phos (Sodium Phosphate); Aquarius – Nat Mur (Sodium Chloride)

SULPHUR – Taurus, Virgo, and Scorpio
Sulphur is essential for healthy hair, skin and nails.
Helps maintain oxygen balance necessary for proper brain function.
Works with B-complex vitamins for basic body metabolism, and is part of tissue-building amino acids.
Aids the liver in bile secretion
No RDA has been set, but a diet sufficient in protein will generally be sufficient in Sulphur.

IN ADDITION
Tones up skin and make hair more lustrous.
Helps fight bacterial infections.

DEFICIENCIES
Unhealthy looking hair.
Brittle hair.

BEST NATURAL FOODS
Lean beef, dried beans, fish, eggs, cabbage.

ZODIAC SIGN
Taurus – Nat Sulph (Sulphate of Soda); Libra – Nat Phos (Phosphate of Soda); Aquarius – Nat Mur (Chloride of Soda or Sodium Chloride)

Planet & Constellation	Tissue Salt by Schuessler
Sun/Leo	Magnesium Phosphate
Mercury/Gemini	Potassium Chloride /Kali Mur
Mercury/Virgo	Sulphate of Potash/Kali Sulph
Venus/Taurus	Sulphate of Soda/Nat Sulph
Venus/Libra	Phosphate of Soda/Nat Phos
Moon/Cancer	Fluoride of Lime/Calc Fluor
Mars/Aries	Potassium/Phosphate
Jupiter/Sagittarius	Silica

Saturn/Capricorn	Phosphate of Lime/Calc Phos
Uranus/Aquarius (table salt)	Chloride of Soda/Nat Mur aka Sodium Chloride
Neptune/Pisces	Phosphate of Lime/Ferr Phos
Pluto/Scorpio	Sulphate of Lime/Calc Sulph

CONSTELLATIONS CELL/TISSUE SALT COMPOSITION

Below is the basic cell structure believed to make up the human body formed by Schuessler in tissue remedies. Separately as indicated the medical field uses the advisedtissue salts but, it needs to be realized that it is the combination of the tissue salts that work the best. In saying that any product used in excess can cause the same problem as seen in insufficient chemical composition, and by doing individual tests on the chemicals mentioned a doctor can restrict or increase as necessary. Separate research has been provided by http sites m.webmed.boots.com - Potassium; victoriahealth.com – Silica;

Areas	Kali	Phos	Mur	Nat	Sulp	Calc	Fluor	Silica	Mag	Ferr	Beneficial Uses
Aries /Mars /1 Skull/Head & Muscles	❁	❁									♈ Potassium Found to strengthen Muscles
Taurus/Venus/2 Neck/Thyroid & Growth Hormone				❁	❁						♉ Natrium is also a Soda i.e. Soda drinks
Gemini/Mercury/ 3 Lungs Nervous & Respiratory System	❁		❁								♊ Mercury in too much quantity found to destroy brain cells
Cancer /Moon/4 Stomach & Digestive System						❁	❁				♋ Calcium used for teeth & whitening
Leo /Sun/5 Heart, Cardiovascular System		❁							❁		♌ Magnesium is used in hospitals for the heart
Virgo/Mercury/6 Intestines & Intestinal System	❁				❁						♍ Mercury found to be a major problem with intestinal problems

Sign / Ruler / House & Body	1	2	3	4	5	6	7	8	9	10	Notes
Libra /Venus/7 Kidneys, Venous System & Urinary Track		✹		✹							♎ Soda. In particular Baking Soda been found to be good for
Scorpio /Pluto/8 Reproduction System					✹	✹					♏ Scorpion not yet researched for reproductive
Sagittarius/Jupiter/ 9 Skin, Liver & Integumentary System								✹			♐ Silica has been found for skin elasticity, hair and nails
Capricorn/Saturn/10 Bones/Knees & Skeletal System		✹				✹					♑ Calcium is known to help Bones
Aquarius/Uranus/ 11 Circulation & Ankles			✹	✹							♒ Chloride and Natrium make up salt needed for circulatory
Pisces/Neptune/ 12 Feet/Lymph		✹								✹	♓ Ferrous is used for lymph problems

Chapter 7 - Gases

Not all planets have gases at least that is what they say, but even the hottest planets will omit some form of gas. Many curers have been brought about by single and combined gases, which I've found to be related to the type of illness related to the planet e.g. Helium is used for respiratory problems and helps to protect the brain tissue. Helium is found in Mercury the planet that rules the respiratory system and the brain

(Ref. Med Gas Res. 2013 Aug – www.ncbi.nlm.nih.gov/m/pubmed/23916029/)

Knowing the right amount for each patient would come down to a specialist in the field or even the specialist performing some experimenting especially for terminally ill people, unfortunately I haven't the facilities to look into this further.

Earth's atmosphere is made up *primarily* of only 2 elements - Nitrogen with 78% and oxygen of 21% as this makes up 99 percent it's obvious all other gases are very minimal.

Hydrogen is very combustible as a pure element mixed with oxygen is what makes water, they state Hydrogen is ruled by Saturn/Capricorn/10th house whilst I've noticed it in a number of planets and Jupiter with 90% in its atmosphere.

Sulphuric Acid is a product formed by the burning of coal and oil the natural product is Sulphur dioxide when omitted into the air it is evaporated by the sun and forms clouds mixed with moisture it's diluted into Sulphuric Acid also known as acid rain.

As we look into gases we find many gases are formed by the burning of metals/minerals and vegetation whatever it may be made up of, makes specific type of gas probably too many to mention.

Carbon Dioxide accounts for 0.03% of the earth's atmosphere and is ruled by Saturn/Capricorn/10th house strangely it takes up half the size of our body in veins.
Nitrogen makes up 78% of earth's atmosphere and is ruled by Uranus/Aquarius/11th house
Oxygen makes up 21% of the air is ruled by Sun/Leo/5th house
Helium ruled by Mercury/Gemini/3rd house
Ether in eyes and spinal canal ruled by Uranus/Aquarius/11th house. Ether is believed to be organic; but, it is also believed to be the outer area of our atmosphere.

Below is a chart of the atmosphere that are surrounding each planet. These could change depending on what literature you read. It could also change depending on the influence of one planet on another when making any type of aspect. This could alter the accuracy of literature we read.

I have found it quite amazing how Carbon Dioxide with such a low percentage has such a powerful impact on earth. 'The atmosphere has increased by more than 40% since the start of the Industrial Revolution, from 280 ppm in the mid-18th century to 402 ppm as of 2016. The present concentration is the highest in at least the past 800,000 years'. (https://en.wikipedia.org/wiki/Carbon_dioxide_in_Earth%27s_atmosphere). One milligram in a kg is 1 ppm (by mass). One liter (L) of pure water at 4°C and 1 standard atmosphere pressure weighs exactly 1 kg, so 1 mg/L is 1 ppm.

Carbon Dioxides is a Saturn influence and under the Encyclopaedia of Medical Astrology states it's a dominant element in earth signs Taurus, Virgo and Capricorn. I'm stating this because it doesn't show up under the cell salts; It causes constraint and retention and Saturn is the main influence in heart attacks. Saturn is known for being a building block building onto one cell after another

	Sun	Mercury	Venus	Earth	Mars	Jupiter	Saturn	Uranus	Neptune	Pluto
Argon		●	●	0.93%	1.60%					
Carbon dioxide		●	96.50%	0.04%	95.32%					●
Carbon Monoxide										●
Helium	7.80%	6%				10%		15.20%	19%	
Hydrogen	92.10%	22%			●	90%	●	82.50%	80%	
Hydrogen Deuteride									192 part /million	
Krypton		●			●					
Methane						●		2.30%	●	●
Neon										
Nitrogen		●	●	78%	2.70%		●			●
Oxygen		42%		21%	0.13%		●			
Radon										
Sulphur/ Sulphuric Acid			●			●				
Water/ Vapour		●	●	0.4 %-1% at Sea	●	●			●	
Xenon		●			●					

	Sun	Mercury	Venus	Earth	Mars	Jupiter	Saturn	Uranus	Neptune	Pluto
Calcium		✿								
Carbon Monoxide					0.08%					
Magnesium		✿								
Potassium		0.50%								
Sodium		29%								
Other				1%						
Ice/ Ammonia							✿	✿		

Ref: www.space.com

Chapter 8 - Working Within the Hours of the Day

This may sound simple but when you compare your own hourly chart you may find yourself working against the celestial hourly chart. This is what I believed happened to me when working on NEVILLE R..'s chart. As soon as I brought something to his attention he wanted me to try it and when I brought to him the hourly system he wanted me to work by it, I did this when doing acupuncture, hypnosis and massage. This I feel you should remember because without a proper analysis it could be psychicly draining. What that meant to me was I was totally exhausted.

Before looking at the planets and the hour they rule let's look at the horoscope, because there are planets that are in their detriment and others that are exalted and so if there is a particular planet that is ruling a particular hour it could be working against you or your client's horoscope if so it could be draining more than instructive. But, who am I to speak, I do everything at the wrong time and I'm still here and my friends have seemed to benefit.☺

Planets in their Detriment, Fall and Exaltation

A planet is said to be in its detriment when it is opposite the sign of its rulership. This causes a planet to be limited in its expression of its basic characteristic.

A planet is said to be in its fall when it's opposite to the sign it is exalted in. When a planet is in its fall it is said to be more hazardous to health.

Planets are strongest in those signs in which they are in their exaltation or rulership. This means they can clearly express the rulership of the planets in that sign. It is good to remember the area of health each planet and constellation rule. For instance, signs in their exaltation i.e. Sun in Aries give thought to the heart and red blood. Moon in Taurus gives thought to stomach/digestive track and throat/thyroid and hormone development. As we continue Mercury in Aquarius gives thought to Brain/Arms/Oxygen/Air and Circulation/Ankles/Electro neurons. Venus in Pisces give thought to Veins/Kidneys/Loin and Lymph system/Feet/clear white cells and antibodies of the body that fight bacteria. Mars in Capricorn gives thought to Red Blood Cells/Blood/Muscles and Bones/Knees. Jupiter in Cancer gives thought to Liver/Blood purifier and Stomach/Digestive track. Saturn in Libra gives thought to Knees/Bones/Vertebrae and Kidneys/Veins. Uranus in Scorpio gives thought to Circulatory system/carrying the oxygen in the blood/ankles and Reproductive Organs/Groin/Hormonal changes. Neptune in Cancer gives thought to Mists/lymph/feet and stomach/digestive track both are water signs so this also adds to the thoughts. As we go on we can extend it to pages if we thought about what each planet and constellation means. I'm just giving the basic structure which if studied individually is very broad. The last in the exaltation is Pluto in Leo, which is the Reproduction Organs/Groin/Gonads and Heart/Blood Circulation.

Detriment	Fall	Exalted
Sun in Aquarius	Sun in Libra	Sun in Aries

Moon in Capricorn	Moon in Scorpio	Moon in Taurus
Mercury in Sagittarius	Mercury in Leo	Mercury in Aquarius
Venus in Scorpio	Venus in Virgo	Venus in Pisces
Mars in Libra	Mars in Cancer	Mars in Capricorn
Jupiter in Gemini	Jupiter in Capricorn	Jupiter in Cancer
Saturn in Cancer	Saturn in Aries	Saturn in Libra
Uranus in Leo	Uranus in Taurus	Uranus in Scorpio
Neptune in Virgo	Neptune in Capricorn	Neptune in Cancer
Pluto in Taurus	Pluto in Aquarius	Pluto in Leo

Now let's look at the Planets and the Hours they rule

First it all begins with a date - 31.7.2001 – the Zodiac sign is Leo, changeover always takes place between 21/22 of each month and lasts till 21/22, an Ephemeris will give you the exact sign if born on the cusp; more importantly for what we are looking at is the exact time the Sun rises and sets; I've always associated Leo with the colour bright yellow but some may say Royal Blue. The zodiac is a proud and noble sign and so people will be more proud and noble than usual throughout the Leo month.

The Day the Planets Rule

The planets flow as follows for week days: -
Sun, Moon, Mars, Mercury, Jupiter, Venus, Saturn and this is fairly easily to remember as the Sun is Sunday, Moon is Monday, Saturn is Saturday and they are 3 names already given you by knowing the planets.

For Tuesday and other days, we need to know a bit of Latin/Germanic or the Nordic mythology as Tiw means Mars and Tuesday came from Tiw/Tyr – Norse god of war, it was Tyrsdag finally it became Tuesday, as such Tuesday is an action day and a good day to begin things.

Wednesday was named after Wodan his role was Father of all Gods, also known as Oden. From Wodan came Wednesday. He had to do with wisdom/ poetry, war and death. He was able to speak to the dead to question the wisest, so it's a communicative day and one of deep thought. It's also ruled by Mercury = Mercurii. God of trade/profit/merchants and travellers, the original trade was in corn.

Thursday was named after Thor god of thunder, one of the most powerful gods. He was said to be protector of gods and humans Thor became Thursday.

Friday was the day named after goddess Frigg wife of Oden/Wodan, patron of marriage/motherhood/love and fertility. This is maybe why we often hear people say I love Fridays.
Ref. Micha F. Lindemans – Encyclopedia Mythica

The Planets Rulership with the Hours in a Day

The hours have a different rulership to the planets that rule the days of the week. It must be remembered this alters for the hours of 24-hour period. It flows Sun, Venus, Mercury, Moon, Saturn, Jupiter, Mars

The days of the week the planets rule are:

Sunday – Sun
Monday – Moon
Tuesday – Mars
Wednesday – Mercury
Thursday – Jupiter
Friday – Venus
Saturday – Saturn

The first hour after Sunrise on a particular day is ruled by its sign of that day, so if it is a Sunday, the Sun will rule the 1st hour after sunrise. The Moon will rule the first hour from sunrise on Monday etc.

The span that is ruled by the planets is found by calculating the time from sunrise to sunset, which alters from month to month, from season to season from zone to zone and don't forget times are adjusted for daylight saving. In this case Sunrise is 5:40 a.m. Sunset was 6:30 p.m. This gives us 12 hours 50 minutes for the whole daylight period on the 31.7.2001, and, so it's not necessarily going to be an even hour. We then divide 12 h 50 m by 12, as 12 hrs rules night and day and equals 24. When we divide 12 h 50 m by 12 it equals 1 hour 4 minutes with 2 minutes over. We'll take it to the nearest minute which will leave 2 minutes over which is why the last time is 18:28 p.m. These are daylight hours, if you want to be more precise you can, it will take it into seconds which would be 5.40.10 a.m. but I'm rounding it off.

We'll begin our week with a Sunday and divide the daylight hours by 12 and therefore each planet will occupy 1 hour and 4 minutes of day light hours.

Please note the change in rulership of hours to those of days.

For Sunday

1st hr ruled by the Sun	5:40 – 6:44 a.m.
2nd hr ruled by Venus	6:44 – 7:48 a.m.
3rd hr ruled by Mercury	7:48 – 8:52 a.m.
4th hr ruled by the Moon	8:52 – 9:56 a.m.
5th hr ruled by Saturn	9:56 – 11:00 a.m.
6th hr ruled by Jupiter	11:00 – 12:04 p.m.
7th hr ruled by Mars	12:04 – 13:08 p.m.
8th hr ruled by Sun	13:08 – 14:12 p.m.
9th hr ruled by Venus	14:12 – 15:16 p.m.
10th hr ruled by Mercury	15:16 – 16:20 p.m.
11th hr ruled by the Moon	16:20 – 17:24 p.m.
12th hr ruled by Saturn	17:24 – 18:28 p.m. Sunset

The nightfall or sunset to sunrise is calculated the same way, sunset I've rounded off to 06:30 p.m. or 18:30 hrs, sunrise is 5:40 a.m. the next day, the interval then is 11 hrs 10 mins, multiply 11 x 60 = 660 minutes + 10 minutes = 670 divide this by 12 this comes to 55.8333 minutes. I've brought it to 56 which puts it out by 2 minutes; 2 minutes multiplied by 60 = 120 seconds / by 12 = -5 seconds for each hour if you want to be precise.

The pattern on the role of planets has already been set by the above calculations for sunrise to sunset, we then continue with the next planet after Saturn ♄ which ruled the last 12th.

As such it would follow for nightfall 6:30 p.m:-

For Sunday
1st hr is ruled by Jupiter   18:30 - 19:26 p.m.
2nd hr is ruled by Mars   19:26 - 20:22 p.m.
3rd hr is ruled by Sun   20:22 - 21:18 p.m.
4th hr is ruled by Venus   21:18- 22:14 p.m.
5th hr is ruled by Mercury   22:14 - 23:10 p.m.
For Sunday / Monday
6th hr is ruled by Moon   23:10 - 00:06 a.m.
7th hr is ruled by Saturn   00:06 - 01:02 a.m.
8th hr is ruled by Jupiter   01:02 - 01:58 a.m.
9th hr is ruled by Mars   01:58 - 02:54 a.m.
10th hr is ruled by Sun   02:54 - 03:50 a.m.
11th hr is ruled by Venus   03:50 - 04:46 a.m.
12th hr is ruled by Mercury   04:46 - 05:42 a.m

An adjustment for the next day begins at Sunrise, if it's Tuesday Mars begin's the first hour at sunrise etc.

By this section you should know the planets meaning; and that this book is a reference book for astrologers. I'm saying that because I'm reflecting on the characteristic of the Sun, when it's not afflicted it brings clarity and it rules the heart, some say it's the expression of the will. If it's afflicted by Mars there can be too much heat especially if Mars is in a fixed sign, remember that Mars rules the red blood cells and the muscles, if it is in a fixed sign of Aquarius which is opposite Leo this is also fixed by it's quadruplicity, you have to remember to look at the house if the Sun is in 7th house we are looking at the person being active. This is where it becomes complex. 7th house is ruled by Libra its quadruplicity is cardinal. Mars in Aquarius would mean it would be stopping the fluids that is pumped by the electrodes in the circulatory system. This is because too much heat with Mars and Sun both fire sign would dry the air or oxygen up in the circulatory system, stopping the electrical pump in the system.

Chapter 9 - Colours

Colours are an important part in finding a cure, and I believe further studies are needed. Satellite images display colours that seem simple; but, they can be distorted by gases, a planet's surface may be red as in Venus whilst with the white clouds it becomes a brown/pink. The Earth appears blue and white because it is believed the water is evaporated into the atmosphere and the white clouds are due to the Sun's action, it doesn't mention the green we presume would be their due to forests and replanting of trees or the brown from the denuding of trees and the green the ocean normally is.

When I look for a formula an important procedure I do is to mix the colours of the constellations and planets and combine the conjuncts, those where another planet is at the same degree or near, I try and imagine what the colour then would be.

In illness there are many areas of discharge, just in the head we have ears, eyes, nose and mouth. In the reproductive area there are the bladder/urinary track, bowel/anus, vagina or penis for men. Whilst men use the same structure for urinary track and sperm, they are two separate structures within one. We also have pores in out body that discharge sweat, we don't think of it having colour but I have seen yellow fluid being released on a body that has just died. There are many different types of infection that changes the colour of the excreted fluids whether it be from your head/reproductive organ or pores it is the colour we are relating to here which we can associate with planets/constellations and even houses.

Colours of planets from satellite images

The old Astrologers who were all Astronomers were thought to not have modern day technology and so the colours they put to planets and constellations were assumed to be from their native eye, observed from earth, but, archaeologists are finding unbelievable instruments in tombs and elsewhere that's hard to explain and in latter times they've found similarities to what was thought to be new inventions to those buried in tombs. I've found conflict in some Astrology site; one in particular is their colour of Libra being green, satellite imagery doesn't agree, as below, and I've found nothing to support it, except the gall bladder and oil it holds is green, as such I believe there are secondary colours.

The Satellite Colours

Mars	red-dark orange caused by rustic rocks.
Mercury	grey, it has no atmosphere and shows the rock surface, but it could also be the colour of mercury.
Venus	pinky brown - the atmosphere is yellowish-white which makes the surface rock red appear pinky brown which was found by the NASA the Magellan project.
Earth	blue, it is the atmosphere caused by the oceans and light where it also can be seen as light blue and white clouds.
Jupiter	orange and white bands, its believed the bands are coloured by ammonia clouds, and the orange comes from ammonium hydro Sulphideide clouds of which the planet is made up.
Saturn	pale yellow, this is caused by white ammonia haze. In the planets winter the northern hemisphere appears blue.

Uranus	light blue, caused by the methane clouds.
Neptune	light blue (yet darker then Uranus), caused by methane clouds.
Pluto	light brown, believed to have dirty methane ice on the surface.

V
The colours of planets I use to depict planets causing illness.
Some colours could be the association of other planets.

Mars	red-orange
Aries	as above
Venus	pale pink, the colour of the venous system mixed with CO^2 - as associated to the Earth Element of Taurus.
Taurus	reddish brown, a dirty red-maroon
Mercury	Mercury's colours change to what planets are affecting it, as such it could be gray contributed to a cloud affect, also the name indicates a deadened gray or silver metallic colour.
Gemini	as above
Moon	white
Cancer	white and black, indication of full moon and new moon.
Sun	yellow-red-mustard
Leo	as above
Mercury	as seen as an earth's colour, mercury silver or deadened gray.
Virgo	as above
Venus	pink
Libra	as above
Pluto	dark purple-dark brown-light maroon, black
Scorpio	as above
Saturn	dark brown/black
Capricorn	brownie black
Uranus	blue, the colour of the sky
Aquarius	as above
Neptune	Mist colour, green of lakes
Pisces	as above

The below show the three initial colours called the primary colour which all other colours come from. Compliments of Google. I'm endeavouring to show how when each colour is mixed with another it can be understood by an astrologer, it is a specialized field so not all would have studied it, in saying that I feel my knowledge is limited, but, there is a lot I have learnt when making formulas and looking for specific colours. Heat changes a colour, water causes colours to be more translucent as do gases, colours mixed with earth gives them a degree of quality.

In astrology dark yellow is the colour of the Sun and ruled by the Sun, Leo and 5th house; blue is the colour of the Sky ruled by Uranus, Aquarius and 11th house. Pink is the colour of Venus, whilst the planet is a red rock the natural gases makes it look pink. If we look at our environment it's the atmosphere which relates to the gases that are transformed by the Sun causing photosynthesis which has brought about the greenery of our forests; where green is seen as a secondary colour.

The colours below are through darkroom filters, I found these interesting because they show black and white, Magenta has been created by red and blue, Cyan has been created by green and blue.

There seem to be a confusion to what the primary colours are, with the transparencies above we see how several colours affect the pure colours if there are such things as pure colours, as primary colours are colours that can't be made by other colours but I would say 4 colours red, blue, green and yellow seem to make more sense to me. This coincides with the findings of Ewald Hering. In astrology the opposites are necessary to make the squaring colour and there isn't a colour that can't be made it's just finding the right mixture.

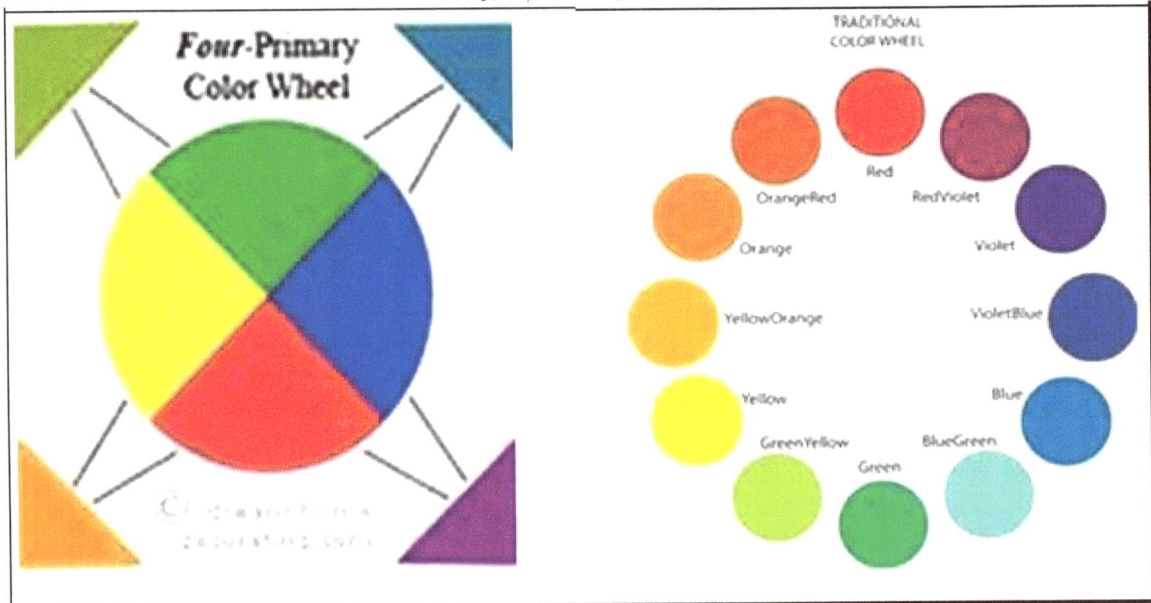

The above is an example of the four primary and colours made from those, found at
http://www.bing.com/images/search?q=images+for+free+of+4+Primary+Colours&id=15834B77D7

42

Primary colours could be more looked upon in astrology as fixed colours.

Water Colours and How They Give a Wishy Washy Affect

The graph above is chart by James Gurney who painted a chart of watercolour pigment combinations. http://gurneyjourney.blogspot.com/2010/10/overlaid-wash-test.html

I've thrown in the water colours because there are 3 water signs/groups and if you're not using a pure chalk like pigment than there is some form of fluid in the paint which adjusts the colour, alcoholic bases are formed by Neptune/Pisces/12th house the other two are Moon/Cancer/4th house and Pluto/Scorpio/8th house these signs rule ocean/lakes/rivers/marshes and mists. Having mentioned Pluto, it made me remember that some painters used to use their own faeces or that of animals, which is manure at least this is what I saw in a documentary and if you think about a painter in the bush they'd need to be inventive to find their colours a few hundred years ago, but I understand it tendered to crack unless there was oil mixed with it. Personally, it wouldn't be a picture I'd seek to buy.

I love these Colours as they are really giving you the watery effect, that can only be seen with the water signs and their rulers. The changes are particularly noticed with the yellow, and how you can see how it changes the pinks and blues. Of course, I relate yellow to the Sun, Blues to the Earth but the paler shades the Sky – Aquarius.

In health a washed out look is often the look which leukemia gives can be contributed to Neptunian problem. An indigo/mauveish. wishy-washy look can often be contributed to Pluto an affect mixed with a paler colour maybe the white of the Moon in such a case one could look to the hormonal structure and stomach problems. I've noticed mottled colours are found in mutable signs i.e. Virgo, Pisces, Gemini and Sagittarius. Mottle colours are those with specks of colour or waves i.e. in clouds. We also see it a lot in horse races.

THE GIRL WITH ACNE

With colours and health problems colours are changed by the influence of other planets, which I've tried to show with the combinations, but if there was a pure colour our body actually tells us by what we see. To explain this, I once treated a girl who came to stay a few days, she had pimples on her face that were unusual, no one had been able to help her and nothing she bought from the supermarket had worked, I began telling her what constellation ruled the head, which is ruled by Aries, it ruled problems with pimples, which are spear shaped and red, its character is to be aggressive, active, but this had to be set off by something. I then explained to her what the cardinal signs meant which involved partnership, family, and constraint it eventually came out that her partner's family, his father in particular was going to be released from prison and had been a child molesterer. Her partner wanted his father to be part of his family, and only 6 months earlier she had given birth to a little boy. She had tried to fight her partner on this, but he said he couldn't do that to his father.

She had a huge decision to make. As she spoke her face was healing. The pimple colour changed so I had to change the treatment to incorporate the new colours. I can only remember the last treatment I gave her, was a pre-prepared food, actually supermarket bought, that combined the colours of blue and white and had been fermented to achieve this, which I asked her to put on the pimples. I looked for a food that had the same action the stomach does, for it has hydrochloric acid in the stomach which ferments its food, this action is ruled by Cancer. The action I took helped her to clear up what I now believe was a type of psoriasis but it wasn't scaly so there could be another name, which I can't find. I put it down to bringing up concerns she hadn't been able to speak about and the treatments I was able to do over the 3 days. When she left she was a much a happier girl and I believe that was due to being able to understand her situation. In my case when the colour of the symptoms changed it meant there was more research to do. By the third night she was not embarrassed to go out. :) The reference book I would have used would have been Encyclopaedia of Medical Astrology by H.L. Cornell M.D. and this is why I've expanded on colours below.

When there are problems and when these colours are seen you can look to these: -
Red is the colour of Mars - health signs: - redness, red skin, rashes, blood hyperactivity, headaches, sudden cuts, anything that appeared spear shaped. The colour relates to problems with actions.
Pink to dark crimson is the colour of Venus or Libra (not Taurus), problems with acid in urine, salt in urine, kidneys and urinary problems, veins, lower back pain. The colour relates to problems with love ones, if Taurus money.
Black is the colour of Saturn/Capricorn: - causes problems with blockages, crystallization, knee pain, black discolouration of the skin shows a blockage in the air flow. The colour relates to problems with government, work, and the older generation.
Yellow to orange is colour the Sun/Leo: - orange discolouration, means there are problems with the heart or oxygen in the blood. The colour relates to problems with entertainment, self and patriarch or son's.
Yellow to light yellow is the colour of Jupiter/Sagittarius and means problems with the liver. The colour relates to problems with philosophies, universities, religion all areas of an overseas nature.

If we complicate matters as below we see what happens with a mixture of colours: -
Magenta/purple is the colour of Venus mixed with the Sun /Leo comes red Aries
Cyan is the colour of Pisces mixed with Magenta Libra makes blue the colour of blue/Aquarius
Cyan Magenta and Yellow are the colours of Pisces/Libra/Leo or Neptune/Venus/Sun = Black
White is the colour of the Moon/Cancer and mixed with Neptune, which makes colours more penetrable, this could be seen in anaemia.

As such we can look at illnesses through colour. If a person has gone blue, they've been deprived of oxygen. Oxygen is pumped to the heart by the lungs it allows our body to puff up, it's an invisible gas and part of the air we consume which contains hydrogen, nitrogen, carbon dioxide. It's a sign that the heart has stopped working. The hearts function is to combine oxygen with blood, the blue veins have carbon dioxide in them which we can see if we put a tourniquet around our upper arm and watch the blue vein come to the surface and sometimes we only need to open our hand and look at our wrist, because it's not a clear colour we'd call it polluted and yet some parts of the body requires carbon dioxide which is brought to them through the mixture of blood and so it's been found that the colour comes from the mixture of carbon dioxide and blood. Ultimately they go to the heart to be cleansed and the arteries take the renewed blood, the red blood around our body, in fact the body has a recycling system. If we look at charts and figurines it looks like it's defined, where red takes over from blue but in fact it isn't. When the body dies the pores release all types of different colours which has been dependent on what we eat. But, there again colours could differ depending on what the illness has taken and what it has   left.

Colour Chart

	Sun Yellow	Mercury Silver	Venus Pale Pink	Earth Blue	Moon White	Mars Red	Jupiter Dirty Yellow	Saturn Brown/ Black	Uranus Light Blue	Neptune Green	Pluto Indigo
Sun											
Mercury											
Venus											
Earth											
Moon											
Mars											
Jupiter											
Saturn											
Uranus											
Neptune											
Pluto											

Illustrations of Colour of Planets when Conjunct

I have created the boxes below using the chart above and adding the colours I've created to show a multi-colour affect, the centre colour is the outcome from it, it's the colour we can expect to see when there is planetary problems causing illness.

Yellow & Black /Sun & Saturn

When we look at the Sun it's generally bright yellow unless other factors have changed it. If it's fire which has turned the sky red, we're looking at Mars/Jupiter & Sun. Here we're looking at Saturn. Saturn blocks oxygen which is ruled by the Sun and without oxygen we die. Going a yellow grey is a colour of lack of oxygen, blockages to the heart are usually a build-up of calcification, these are calcium blocks/cells built on top of each other, the building of something is a Saturn influence but, calcium is part of its cell salt.

Pink & Yellow - Sun & Venus

Venus's colour is that of red rock covered by a cloud which makes it pink/brown. It is the colour for both Taurus and Libra. Whilst veins are ruled by Libra under the Venous System the colour of varicose veins is an actual adulteration of the natural colour of Venus and shows the lack of oxygen, but If we have the Sun and Venus together we are likely to see a pale orange. You could find a heated thyroid or heated kidneys if there are problems. Taurus and Libra have a natural health problem aspect if there are planets in those signs, but usual this isn't the case, only one other are shared by the same planet.

Blue & Yellow - Sun & Earth
The Earth has been called the water planet as is illustrated by blue, and whilst the Sun is always in the opposite sign to the Earth if there are additional problems and the fluids of the body are being affected we get the grey/yellow colour, much like that of varicose veins. A lighter mix of yellow and blue stands for circulation problem under which would be seen with Uranus.

Grey & Yellow - Greeny Blue - Jupiter/Mercury - Neptune
Here the colours become more complicated Jupiter and Mercury is the colour of Grey and Yellow mixed this gives the combined colour as seen in the Colour Table above when it's added to Neptune it becomes a smokey greeny/blue/brown which is the centre colour. Neptune does have a smokey/misty affect.

ANATOMY AND THE ZODIAC

This shows the relationship between the Zodiac and the Anatomy and the special relationship between the signs and the body. Often illness comes from polarity of the opposite sign, e.g. Aries – Libra, if there is a headache it could be related to a kidney problem ruled by Libra.

Aries - Libra
Aries rules the head, they often suffer headaches. The glands are the subrenals, beneath the kidneys, which pumps adrenalin into the blood for emergencies

Taurus – Scorpio
Taurus rules the throat and neck. They are particularly vulnerable to colds and chills. The gland is the Thyroid any problems will lead to weight problems

Leo – Aquarius
Leo rules the heart, spine & back. They have a tendency to enjoy themselves too much, they need to slow down as they get older for heart problems

Gemini – Sagittarius
Gemini rules the nerves arms and shoulders. Their prone to break collar-bones and arms. Internally lungs where colds often turn into bronchitis. Gemini's are restless live on their nerves.

Libra – Aries
Libra rules the kidneys any disruption to their lives can result in a back pain relating to the kidneys.

Cancer - Capricorn
Cancer rules the stomach, mammary glands and alimentary canal. Their tendency is to get upset and worry more than most. They're prone to indigestion and ulcers.

Scorpio – Taurus
Scorpio rules the sexual organs. They are more highly sexed then other signs. Any frustration or suppression can lead to unpleasant behaviour.

Virgo – Pisces
Virgo rules the nervous system and intestines; they suffer from bowel & stomach problems. They can be worriers due to nervous tension

Capricorn – Cancer
Capricorn rules the knees, bones and teeth. Orthopaedic and dental troubles are common as with deterioration of the bones.

Sagittarius – Gemini
Sagittarius rule the liver, hips and thighs. Sagittarius stagnate if they don't give themselves considerable amount of mental and physical exercise resulting in excessive weight.

Pisces – Virgo
Pisces rules the Lymph system and the feet. As such they should always wear well fitted shoes, with a common ailment being anaemia.

Aquarius – Leo
Aquarius rules circulation and ankles. They can suffer from varicose veins and hardening of the arteries. Fractures are common in the shin and ankles

ANATOMY AND THE PLANETS

This gives a brief outline of the planets relationship over the endocrine glands that release hormones into the blood.

Mercury
Mercury is associated with the respiration, the brain and the nervous system which gives strong links to all parts of the body.

Venus
Venus rules the throat, kidney, lumbar and parathyroid. These play an important part in controlling the calcium levels in the body.

The Sun
The Sun rules the heart, back and spinal column, and assoc. with the thymus, an endocrine gland behind the upper end of the sternum that is important to puberty. With a connection between the immunization against bacteria.

The Moon
The Moon is connected with the breasts and the whole alimentary, or food system - the oesophagus, stomach, liver, gall bladder, bile ducts, pancreas and intestines.

Jupiter
Jupiter has always been linked with the biggest gland, the liver, and it's purifying function. We now find a strong relationship to the pituitary gland. It regulates hormone production & governs physical growth.

Uranus
Uranus is connected to the circulatory system, the gonads and the pineal body – an area of the brain important to primeval animals, but disputed by man. It's sometime called the 'third eye'.

Pluto
Pluto is linked with Mars in influencing the gonads. It's special connection is with the formation of cells and the reproduction function itself.

Saturn
Saturn is connected with the gall-bladder, spleen, skin, teeth and bones. This later effect is strengthened by its influence on the anterior lobe of pituitary, which relates to the sex glands, bone and muscle structure

Mars
Mars acts upon the muscular and urogenital system and upon the gonads or sex glands – ovaries or testes.

Neptune
Neptune acts upon the general nervous system and in particular the Thalamus – a structure in the brain that gives a vital part in the transmission of stimuli to and from the sensory organs.

Chapter 10 - Example of How Charts Give You The Avenue & Procedure for Formulas

I've given other formula's in the chapter below, the graph below is a simplified version as how I look for formula's. The symptom is a **fixed rash** on the **hips**. Once you understand the meaning of the planets, constellation and houses you go to doing a graph for each of them, taking particular notice to the areas that have close degrees, usually I find quincunx's causing an underlining problem. But with the aspects below we can see what could be a problem if other aspects are affecting it. The aspects I've given if unaffected would probably be just felt as heat and moisture around the liver area and that's where the Quadruplicities and Triplicities come in. When I go by the Encyclopaedia of Medical Astrology it uses all aspects – a rash would be caused by Aries/1st house/Mars which rules pimples; sudden eruptions would be caused by Uranus and hips are the sign of Sagittarius/9th house or Jupiter. If we look at the clients chart we'd look to the areas that we have concluded to be affected by the planets/constellations and houses.

From what we know Mars is a Fire sign, and refers to red, the 9th house is ruled by Sagittarius or Jupiter it's anatomy are the hips/liver, and its colour is dirty yellow, when we combine red and yellow together we get orange, and so the immediate food I thought of was a carrot. The carrot has the shape of a spear. Purple is the colour for the Scorpio constellation which is a fixed sign; as such we could be looking for a purple carrot, as it's covered by the Scorpio influence and relates to the physical appearance on how Mars is depicted, spear shaped. Finally, rice, rice again is spear shaped and it has the expansive qualities of the 9th house renowned for its elasticity, along with Jupiter and Sagittarius rules the skin which is expansive, covering all parts of the body; and, able to renew itself with the help of the immune system, as does the liver which the 9th house and Sagittarius rule, the cell salt for this area is silica which could also be used/this reminds me I've also bought liver for remedies of 9th house etc.

When you decide on what products are used, for confirmation I'd confer with Runes; Now to preparation - we see Mars is a fire sign and Scorpio is a water sign and the 9th house is another fire sign. Those in the fire signs are the orange carrot and the rice, the orange carrot needs to be dried with heat and so it could be fried or grilled, a little bit of history tells us that rice is dried in the Sun and so it has already undergone one of the processes. The purple carrot needs to be prepared by boiling which combines the effect of Mars and leave it to be soured, a property of Scorpio, and an acid. Finally, we combine them after leaving the purple carrot to sour and straining.

The below wouldn't need to be done if there wasn't some planet / aspect affecting it.

Chapter 11 Explanation to Formulas & Examples of Formulas Created

PATIENT – MARK S. PERSON IN A COMA

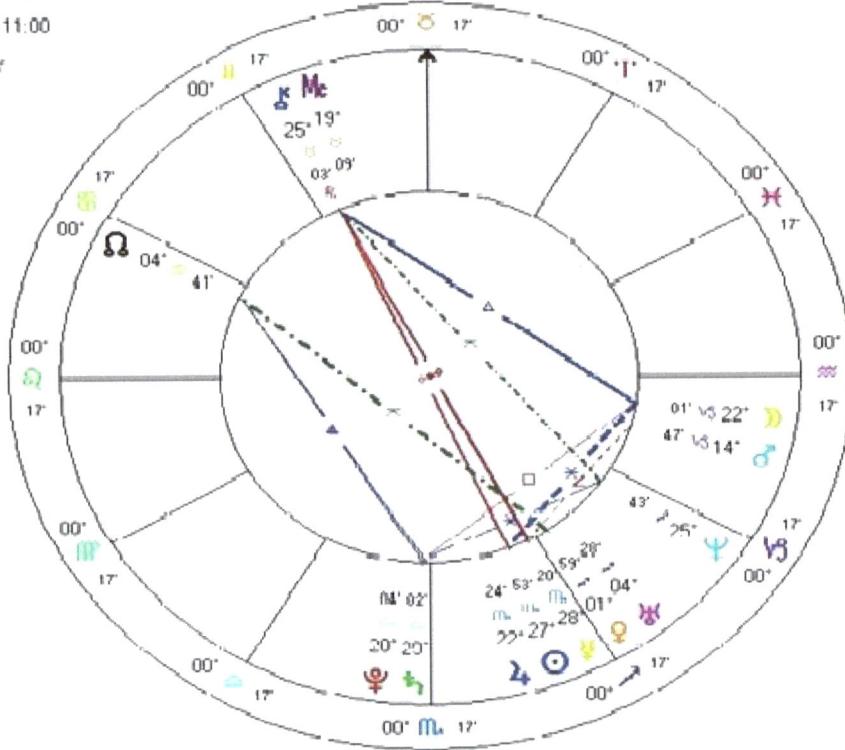

M. S.
Natal Chart (618)
21 Nov 1982
0:05 am AEDT -11:00
Sydney, NSW
33°S52 151°E13'
Geocentric
Tropical
Equal
True Node

Chart 4

Above is the Natal Chart of Mark when he was 29 he had an accident whilst in a televised competition, which left him in a coma, to this day I believe he's still in that coma.

I'm showing the calculations in the chart that led me to several formulas; it would take a whole lot of guts to trial it. But, I've tried so many of my own formulas that work on a usually prolonged temporary basis, as planets change, that I was confident in making it up. Whilst I had reservations in giving his wife the process in which I found the formula, knowing it would only be useful for him as it is based on his personal data for time, date & place for the Natal, Transit & Progressed Charts. I felt I had to give her something as she had paid me $600 for the consultation. If you look at my chart you will see I have a lot of Pisces influences either by Pisces itself or Neptune, but not so much the 12th house, and there are quite a lot of blockages; and this is what causes me problems in doing quantities of analysis'. With Mark It was an innate feeling I had, that I had to get started on formulas. I am at no way confident when having to put to a guardian something has to be digested especially when it smells like something regurgitated, whilst I'd do it to myself if required. As you can imagine the case was quite challenging, and the formulas I've suggested are individual to the client and I had problems giving his wife what I'm about to give you as you can imagine it's my intellectual property, and at some time could be used for someone else, I hope that anyone using my procedures will accord me all rights warranted as having the intellectual property of the forethought.

For myself I had to have the proof that reasoning was correct and at the interview the wife and mother wanted me to see him whilst I was determined not to. In our consultation I brought to them the areas I'd found prominent in his chart. The thing was if I'd seen him they could have said my analysis was based on what I saw. I've always said that astrology was a science based on the planets and stars where you only need an accurate date of birth to begin; with preferably the correct time of birth all else follows, below is what I explained to them. The formulas were never given to him because one in particular smelt extremely bad, it took the longest time to prepare because it had to be fermented. I also suggested that they talk to the head doctor about what I'd found and about the formulas I felt would be required. Below is a detailed outline on what I saw and why I created the several formulas I made. You will see that I've been selective on what aspect I've used and only required the family to act in keeping Mark cool especially around the Transiting period outlined in bold. When looking at the digestion of the fermented crab for his stomach, even though it would have been feed through a tube into his stomach, afterwards I wondered if I could have made into an oil rub.

M. S.
D.O.B. 21 Nov 1982 T.O.B. 0:05 am
Place – Sydney Australia
Progressed date - 27 Nov 2012

The following is giving explanations to how I saw the body malfunctioning with referring to medical astrology, and the planets, constellations and house basics along with there aspect.

Explanation

From M.S's charts I explained what I saw and that was the hormones were being heated causing the groin to be hot, and one of the problems was the hydrochloric acids of the stomach where blocked by the circulatory system, the circulatory system are the fluids carried through the body it involves the electrical system but is prevalent in the intestines. It also showed that groups were upsetting his mind, and that there would be some sign of this physically.

Astrological Explanation
1. Natal Sun 27° Scorpio Square Progressed Moon 24° Aquarius 6th house
The Sun in Scorpio means the hormones are being heated and causing the area to be hot in the groin, what is squaring this area by progression is the Moon, which is moist has to do with the Hydrochloric Acids of the stomach being blocked in the Circulatory System ruled by Aquarius. The Moon is ill placed in Aquarius in the 6th house (a talkative house) meaning family in groups could be physically and mentally, upsetting him, therefore, preferably only 1 or 2 persons at a time. The Moon also rules wives, mother's family and the emotions, physically the stomach and mammary glands. Aquarius rules Groups, the Circulatory system and the Electrical nerves, therefore -

Suggested action
Restricting visitors to 1 or 2.

Explanation

Mark's liver was acting unpredictably in purifying his blood this would cause his skin to appear blue and yellowish and there could be breathing problems because of the focus being on the stomach. It also appears that the hydrochloric acids are having a negative effect on the Liver.

Astrological Explanation

2. Natal North Node 4° 04 in Cancer Quincunx Uranus 06° 17 in Sagittarius
This means that the Liver ruled by Sagittarius is acting unpredictably because of the planet Uranus, Sagittarius also rules the skin/liver would cause the skin to appear blue and yellowish. The stomach could appear white with North Node in Cancer. Sagittarius works against the action of the brain for it naturally opposes Gemini, which is an air sign requiring oxygen. The Cancer sign being 4° prior to the progressed Uranus shows that the hydrochloric acid is playing negatively on the liver. North Node acts much the same way as Sagittarius it expands everything and makes it noticed and so I put a Silica bases to it. The Cancer sign normally makes a 150° aspect to Sagittarius these influence is affected when there are planets in them, any 150° aspects are usually underlying problems.

Suggested formula
Calcium Ferr is what I see in Shell of Crabs. Primarily the Crab is the symbol of Cancerians, I suggest it to be rubbed on ankles which is ruled by Uranus, the Blue Crab which has a blue claw – I've found cooked at Shellharbour Fisheries, can be grinded together keep refrigerated. The blue is the colour for Uranus and i imagine the claw as the ankles of the crab having a relationship to the colour

Explanation
There could be too much attention paid to the stomach whilst the muscles in the circulatory system which bring fluids to the heart and around the heart are becoming fixed. Potassium would be going into the ankles causing them to heat up and possibly causing cramping. The circulatory system requires salt and in fact contrary to popular belief salt helps the stomach produce hydrochloric acid, how it's administered is found in suggestions.

Astrological Explanation
3. Natal North Node in Cancer 4° deg. 04 12th house quincunx Progressed Mars 8° deg. Aquarius in 5th house
North Node in Cancer means attention is drawn to the stomach but what mightn't be obvious is the muscles Mars influence in the circulation is causing problems to the heart 5th house, this would be with salts going into the stomach. Also it could mean too much water in the ankles and a warmth caused through Potassium being focused in the ankles heating up the Circulatory System.

Suggested formula
Acupuncture around the ankles could help. Mars rules needles. And, as the patient can't talk, where there is excessive heat placing an acupuncture needle in that area would help the potassium's move. If a family member is doing it they'd need to feel for indentations and only

5mm and should be kept away from bone areas.   This can happen anytime family members are there. This could also be performed around the ankle as it's ruled by Aquarius.

Explanation
There is an obvious obstruction where the sugars of the body are causing the stomach not to act effectively, causing calcification around the knees and in the bones

Astrological Explanation
4. Progressed North Node 4 deg 15 Cancer 10th house Opposite Progressed Venus 09 deg 08' Capricorn 4th house
Cancer sign rules the stomach it's an active sign when there is a planet opposing the North Node it shows that planet to be acting untimely being affected by the South Node and in this case it is Venus in Capricorn – Venus implies sugar a carbohydrate is causing the stomach not to act properly. Sugar is ruled by Venus and is likely to cause calcification when the planet is in Capricorn. An interesting comment was made by the mother regarding his legs cramping is in the final notes.

Explanation
The brain requires massage; the brain not being massaged would mean there could be air in the bones that are not being released.

Astrological Explanation
5. Progressed Mercury 14° Capricorn
Mercury rules the brain; Capricorn is an active sign and would mean working in a physical sense. It also could mean that there is too much air in the bones, and possibly the Marrow of the bones. Mercury being an air sign. Capricorn ruling the ligaments/bone/knees and marrow inside the bone it is also a cardinal/active sign which differs from Mercury which is mutable/talkative and air sign.

Suggested action
Massaging around the head should be beneficial, as the head is covered by bone and is continually rejuvenating itself massaging should help to promote the air through the bone structure. The other area that could benefit with massaging are the knees. An alternative could be putting air on the knees for brief periods

Explanation
There can be seen infection, if red and heat can be felt in the bones where acupuncture could help, it's caused through heat of the blood affecting the calcium of the bones and minerals and the marrow unable to reproduce, for suggested treatment refers to suggested formula.

Astrological Explanation
6. Natal Mars in Capricorn
Mars is in its detriment in Capricorn it can mean being aggressive in the field of work, where Capricorn is already an active sign and not one to sit on its laurels. This involves heat in the bone structure.   It can mean that the Marrow in the Bone is heating and therefore the natural regeneration of the bone system is having problems rejuvenating itself, Mars also rules the Blood and it's action of using the muscles gets the blood flowing, this will be another area needing to be looked at, but the treatment below intends to help this problem.

Suggested formula
   a.   Recommended formula - Time: 9 – 10 Tuesday Best day to work on muscles.
¼ tspn of Crushed Wheat an earth/air mix with 1 tspn of Hot Chilli Sauce this needs to be rubbed into the back of the head – Cerebrum and Cerebellum
b.   This aspect shows acupuncture on the head at the Chinese meridian Du 20 useful. I'm suggesting only one needle, which a family member could learn to do, laying the needle flat facing horizontally between each ear. (It's the last area to mend in the head as a child) where there is an indentation in the top of the head, I have provided diagrams to show how to find meridian points. Ex 6 meridians actually circles the area in the top of the head, Ex 6 point can be used after you see a reaction. You could also place heated wheat around the knees.

Astrological Explanation
7. Planets in the House position affecting the Brain – Best day to work on Kidneys is Friday
3rd House aspects Natal Pluto 28° deg. 04 Libra

Pluto in Libra means an excess amount of sugar in the Kidneys.   This would mean the Kidneys would be finding it hard to get rid of the Sulphates It could be also depleting the air to the kidneys. Bringing this to the doctor's attention as patient could inhale a very minute amount of nitrogen, which is a substance of Pluto's

Transiting Jupiter in Gemini 21-1- 13
For this day it shows the influence of Jupiter possibly expanding the air in the lungs. These are areas that need to be monitored by a doctor.

Suggested formula
a Inhaling Nitrogen .5 mm alternately 3 drops of Ammonia in 2 tbspn of Saline, 2 tbspns of water in Asthma machine, probably be all that's needed.

Astrological Explanation
Transiting Mars 20° 03 in Aquarius squaring Jupiter 22° 24 in Scorpio
This aspect for a few days around 21-1-13 will need to be kept an eye on.
this can mean that the Air to the Brain is heated and could at times be blocked by being dried out with too much heat, and constant monitoring should take place.

Suggested action
a. A damp cloth on the Brain and temporal area recommended.

Explanation
There could be seen calcification or excessive calcium in the kidneys.

Astrological Explanation
Saturn 29° Libra 3rd house.
d) Saturn is a planet which is naturally working when in Libra it can be found that it works against the action of the kidney, doctors will probably find the kidney working too hard.

Suggested action

a. Saturn in Libra shows a Potash or crushed Calcium Phosphate they are ruled by Saturn, and would probably be useful on the Kidneys as this planet would be probably restricting the Air both in the kidneys and lungs and required action to the Brain. Using the above could breakdown the Calcification that has been built up. A form of Air Brushing would be best for the kidney area and massaging it into the Lung area.

Explanation
The blood from the liver could be forced into the groin instead of kidneys and bone marrow.

Astrological Explanation
8. Natal and Progressed (N/P) Jupiter in Scorpio in 4th house
Jupiter rules the liver whilst Scorpio rules the reproductive organs, the 4th house is normally that of Cancer which rules the stomach this shows the purified blood has been forced into the groin instead of the kidneys and bone marrow, which is used to rejuvenate the bone. Resulting with problems with the stomach.

MOTHER AND WIFE'S INFORMATION

In the consultation the areas I focused on caused them to inform me that he was being intravenously fed through his stomach and so there was a lot of focus on his stomach. I stated he was getting upset with crowds and his mother said he appeared agitated at visiting times. I said in his own way he was talking and his mother said 'yes, he made murmurs'. When I said there were problems with his knees they informed me that he'd recently had surgery on his hamstring because his knees were cramping up.

M. S.   Accident
D.O.B. 21 Nov 1982   18 July 2011
0:05 am   9.05 am
Sydney

Combined Aspects of Natal and Transits show problems that occurred at time of accident should be compared to progression

Natal / PLANETS in GREEN at the time of the Accident

PLANET	DEGREE/Min	CONST	HOUSE	ASPECT	PROGRESSED
Sun	27° 63'	Scorpio	4		
Pluto	28° 04'	Libra	3		
Mercury	28° 20'	Scorpio	4		
Saturn	29° 02'	Libra	3	Saturn 150deg	
Neptune	00° 26'	Pisces	7	Neptune	
Venus	01° 59'	Sagittarius	5		
Uranus	04° 28'	Sagittarius	5		
Uranus	04° 32'	Aries	8	Uranus square	
Nth Node	04° 41'	Cancer	12	Nth Node	
Sth Node	04° 41'	Capricorn	6	& Sth Node	Sth Node 04° 15'
Pluto	05° 43'	Capricorn	6	Nth Node oppos.	Capricorn sq Uranus
Jupiter	07° 25'	Taurus	9	Pluto conj Sth Node	Uranus 06° 17'
Saturn	11° 26'	Libra	2	Jupiter 150°	Jupiter sq Mars 8° Aquarius

57

Mars _____ 14° 47'	Capricorn	6	Saturn square	Venus 9° 42'
Venus _____ 16° 54	Cancer	12	Mars; Mars opp	Capricorn sq Saturn
_____			Venus	in Libra
Mars _____ 18° 50'	Gemini	11		Mercury 14° 45'
Mercury _____ 21° 43'	Leo	1		Capricorn sq Venus
Moon _____ 22° 01'	Capricorn	6		
Jupiter_____ 22° 24'	Scorpio	4		
Nth Node _____ 23° 06'	Sagittarius	5		
Sun _____ 25° 02'	Cancer	12		
Neptune_____ 25° 13'	Sagittarius	6		
Moon _____ 26° 40'	Aquarius	7		

M. S., 21 Nov 1982 - Progressed 27 Nov. 2012 Flow Chart

	Deg	Const	Hse	Quad	Tripl	Area	Area	Negative Aspects	Conj	
Sun	28° 20	Sag	4	Fixed	Fire	Heart	Liver Hips		Nept in Sag /Sun in Sag	Lymp/feet Liver
Jupiter	28° 52	Scor	3	Mut	Fire			NN - Can 210	Pl in Lib / Sat in Lib	
Pluto	28° 59	Libra	2	Fixed	Water			Mars in Aq		NN Liver
Saturn	02° 01	Libra	2	Card	Earth					Cancer 10ʰ dried Milk
NN	04° 15	Cancer	10			Liver	Stomach	NN - Can 150	Ven in Cap/Mercury in Cap	Mars in Aq 6th
SN		Cap	4					Ur - Sag		Wheat air grown
Uranus	06° 17	Sag	3	Fixed	Air					
Mars	08° 02	Aqua	5	Card	Fire			NN in Cancer opp Ven in Cap		NN Liver minced in water
Venus	09° 42	Cap	4	Fix/card	Ea/air					Cancer 10ʰ dried Milk
Mercury	14° 51	Cap	5	Mut/mut	Air/Ea					Ur - iodized Salt
Moon	24° 19	Aqua	6	Card	Water			Saturn in Libra sq Ven in Cap		Sag in 3ʳᵈ Liver air dried
Neptune	26° 49	Sag	4	Mut	Water					Sat - Flour Lib - Strawberries Ven Cap - Oil

When looking at ingredients the foods required are only those where there has been conflict within the planets/houses or constellations, whilst every sign has a food, Sagittarius might be the hardest, but many forms of nuts have silica in them but, I've always found Liver the anatomy part it rules the best.

Below I've expanded on the above as each constellation/house and planet are a part of a triplicity/quadruplicity and are either alkaline or acidic, this is an extension of the first chart I gave, but using the flow chart of the above based on the degrees and minutes, you will find that some planets are seconds apart, and is a consequence of having the correct time. Below helps with colours when cooking, refer to Color Chart for Constellations, House & Planet Color, obviously equally important is whether something should be alkaline or acid, if a product isn't naturally acid or alkaline it may need to be fermented or made into an alkaline and sweetened down, but remember whilst I have every planet/house and constellation there we are only looking for the health aspects that are conflicting with the charts

Constellations	Quad	Trip	Alk	Acid	Hse	Quad	Trip	Planet	Quad	Trip
Sagittarius	Mut	Fire	Alk		4	Card	Water	Sun	Fixed	Fire
Scorpio	Fixed	Water		Acid	3	Mut	Air	Jupiter	Mut	Fire
Libra	Card	Air	Alk		2	Fixed	Earth	Pluto	Fixed	Water
Libra	Card	Air	Alk		2	Fixed	Earth	Saturn	Card	Air
Cancer	Card	Water		Acid	10	Fixed	Card	Nth Node		
Sagittarius	Mut	Fire	Alk		3	Mut	Air	Sth Node		
Aquarius	Fixed	Air	Alk		5	Fixed	Fire	Uranus	Fixed	Air
Capricorn	Card	Earth		Acid	4	Card	Water	Mars	Card	Air
Capricorn	Card	Earth		Acid	5	Fixed	Fire	Venus	Fix/Card	Air/Ea
Aquarius	Fixed	Air	Alk		6	Mut	Earth	Mercury	Mut/Mut	Air/Ea
Sagittarius	Mut	Fire	Alk		4	Card	Water	Moon	Mut	Water
Sagittarius	Mut	Fire	Alk		4	Card	Water	Neptune	Mut	Fixed

Below is another chart combining the transits at the time I spoke with Mark's mother and wife, with the progressions at the time of the accident with the natal chart.

T – Transit P – Progressed □ - Square N – Natal Opp – Opposite.

M.S. Transits/ Progressions and Natal Charts showing Aspects				
Transit (T) 21/01/2013	Aspect	Progress (P) 27/11/2012	Aspect	Natal (N) 21/11/1982
				Sun 27° 53' Scor
				Pluto 28° 04' Lib
		Sun 28° 20' Sag	Nept ♂ Sun	Merc 28° 20' Scor
		Jup 28° 51' Scor	30° P Jup/ N Mercury	
		Pluto 28° 59' Lib	Plu ♂ Sat	Sat 29° 04' Libra
Sun 0° 36' Aqua	Sun □ Jup T			
Nep 1° 40' Pisces	□ N Ven ♈			Ven 1° 59 Sag
Merc 02° 00 Aqua	P Saturn	Sat 2° 01' Libra	□ NN	
	♈ NN	NN 04° 15 Cancer	♈ N NN	Ur 04° 58' Sag
	N NN □ Ur		♂ P Ven	NN 04° 41' Cancer
Ur 05° 13' Aries	□ P Venus			Ur 06° 17' Sag
Jup 06° 30' Gem	Opp P Ur	Uran 06° 17 Sag		
		Mars 08° 02 Aqua		
		Ven 09° 42 Cap		
Pluto 10° 00' Cap				
Saturn 10° 47' Scor				
Ven 14° 12' Cap		Merc 14° 51' Cap		Mar 14° 47' Cap
Moon 17° 00 Taur	♂ N Jup			
	□ T Mn/T Mars			
Mars 20° 03 Aqua	□ T Mars//Jup		□ NP Jupiter	Mn 22° 01 Cap
	□ T Mars/T NN			Jup 22° 24 Scorpio
NN 23° 47 Scor	□ P Moon			
		Mn 24° 19 Aqu	□ NP Jupiter	
		Nept 26° 49' Sag		Nep 25° 43' Sag

Chart 5

N.R Natal Chart

7 Nov 1943
6.30 pm AEDT -11:00
Mudgee. NSW
32°S36' 149°E35'
Geocentric
Tropical
Equal
True Node

The above Astrology Chart is the Natal Chart of a person who had a stroke either playing or after playing football, his age was around 27, at the time of volunteering for astrology formulas he was 59. Over a 3-day period with following the Natal, Progress and Transit great progress was made where the therapy he received was gentle but proved strong, at the end of three days he was almost walking with both feet on the ground, his posture had improved and every month he improved more, it lasted 15 months when a lump on the other ankle appeared, unfortunately I wasn't consulted, but I did have a feeling that a negative reaction would come about when I saw him embarrassed and abused at his favourite club, after all he'd been paralysed the left side of his body for 32 years.

When we first started the therapy I needed to explain to him that I didn't know how his body would react because in Astrology in medicine there are four major concerns which relate to signs that are opposite and squaring each other concerning an illness, this has been supported over and over again by the medical profession, and, because I didn't have a computer mind I wouldn't know what would happen in a months or a years' time, but, I stressed if he had any problem he had to tell me, and so I explained the opposite and squaring signs Neville R. would need to be

60

aware of. As a Scorpion his sign ruled the reproductive areas, opposite is Taurus which rules the Thyroid/throat and neck, squaring is Leo which rules the heart, and Aquarius which rules the circulation and ankles. Maybe I just didn't emphasis enough. As he was a Scorpion I was scared as he had 8 areas in fixed constellations and houses. As they were in fixed areas I felt the organ may have shrivelled up with the enzymes not getting to them. I explained that I believed that the strain of an organ suddenly working could affect any of these opposing and squaring areas, and that I wanted him to tell the doctor what we had done, and, what changes he found in himself.

He admitted years later he thought it was a game.

Unfortunately, when I again saw him I'd put myself into a bad financial dealing and I was over stressed and not handling things very well. Where my word came over all common sense and self-preservation, in fact nothing was making sense, I had still been trying to get formulas reviewed by Ministers and just as Neville R. had told me he thought working with astrology was stupid I believe that's what I thought Ministers were thinking. Later I explained to him that the 3 days we spent over the Easter Weekend I'd put my heart and soul into it. I was working on hours in his chart, when to do the acupuncture, the massage, and I was making up formula's on the spot. I was buying the foods that I had no money for, because I wanted to help him. I'd also explained to him that I had taken many a formula to a Minister and asked for reviews, where they would be forwarded to the government research department, to only find two years later they were patented. Throughout my life I was plagued with computer problems and when I'd addressed the Minister for copies of my letters they were appropriately lost.

What I couldn't understand is why Doctors didn't know how to treat a lump on a limb, which could only be fluid and so he reverted to limping. He said 'he couldn't afford to have his good leg fail him'.

The sudden abuse he had at the local bowls club, would be seen in his chart by possibly a Mercury /Uranus aspect or an associated form. There can already be seen quincunxes with Uranus in Gemini 7° 2nd house and Mercury in Scorpio 12° 7th house. To be convinced a progressed & transit chart would need to be added to his natal, where I've done an estimated progress below.

The situation was he was showing me how to play bowls when he was abused, which leads me to Uranus. unpredictable and Mercury rules the neighbourhood. In checking the transits whilst it can't be exact 15 months later Mercury was conjunct Uranus and as the progress Sun moves 1 day a year it would be making health problem by a quincunx aspect. As such this shows how treatment can be altered and how astrologers can look to future aspects, for altering formulas.

Now to the formulas, as always the formulas are made up to find the food types, suggestions can be seen under Foods in this book. For Neville R. a few were pre-prepared and fungi was made when I saw Pisces had planets opposing, surprisingly I'd made these for myself and was amazed I could use them. The therapy itself was on the spare of the moment, and other treatment included alcohol/massage/ hypnotherapy/acupuncture and colour, all of these were based on aspects. It was the first major therapy I had done which required him to keep close contact with his doctor. To see him walk straight brought unexpected jubilation.

Below is the important part of analysing what is required for a formula.

To begin this, I do the *flow chart*. As with Mark it's in order of degrees, you can begin anywhere but I begin with those closest to the Sun. Whenever deciding on colour I've tried to combine the colour of not only the planet but their house and Constellation and the aspects of close planets. Please see 'Colours' for more explanation. This chart helps to see immediately what planets are close to each other. In charts I look to conjuncts with 3°- 6° orbs as with aspects 0°, 90°, 180°, and 150° angles. As with Mark I've done the 3 calculations with Natal, Progress and Transiting, remember that transiting planets are fast moving planets and may only last a short time. The further out planets of course last a lot longer and I usually don't double up because e.g. Pluto may have only moved if 1 degree. The transits must be paid attention to as the formula must be altered once the planets moved on and that food type taken out.

In the flow chart I've repeated the Triplicities and Quadruplicities, these are important in deciding on a colour and way of cooking or preparing the formula. A fire sign indicates orange/yellow and red, and on an obvious level - heat. This is easily seen with a lighter, the top flame is yellow the deeper flames are orange and red, there is always a deeper analogy because when I lit the flame I saw the base of the flame was blue (blues the opposite colour to yellow under Colours, and something has to cause a spark which is the gas and the friction) without air, nothing would be set alight, you wouldn't have a flame at least in the lighter but the flint is another additive. In astrology yellow and blue are fixed colours, they are also known as primary colours along with red and green again refer to Colours. Fixed elements are part of the Quadruplicities and this makes me to believe in the primary colours there are four, not 3 as believed.

In health the fire signs cause a temperature. If there is a blockage in a fire sign the homeostasis of the body would become unbalanced, homeostasis is the regulation of the temperature & enzymes; it means the body wouldn't be able to keep warm or possibly the opposite extreme heat this depends on degrees and whether the planet's degrees are before or after.

Remember he was fine till the aspects 27 years later the flow chart is based on his Natal because this doesn't change, the Progress chart is based on the day month and year and hour we began his treatment. The only foods I'd require for a formula are those making a quincunx, square □, or opposition. There is also the problem of planets being in detrimental signs which they are normally opposite/square ore quincunx which I've also outlined.

Neville R. Flow Chart for D.O.B.

Planets	Deg	Trip	Quad	Acid/	Hse	Trip	Quad	Acid/Alkal.	Const	Trip	Quad	Acid/Alkal.	Aspects	Color	Food
Mercury	12°04	Air	Mut	Alk	7th	Air	Card	Al/Ac	Scor	Water	Fix	Acid	Ur ⚹ Merc Pluto/Leo □Merc/ Scor	Purple	Celery/Air, Polluted cooked Drink water
Moon	12° 31	Water	Card	Acid	11th	Air	Fixed	Alk	Pisces	Water	Mut	Acid		White/Blue	
Sun	14° 01	Fire	Fixed	Alk	7th	Air	Card	Al/Ac	Scor	Water	Fix	Acid	Sn/Mars	Yellow/Red, Yellow/Black	Tomatos Cooked with seed + Hot Sauce
Mars	21° 29R	Fire	Card	Alk	2nd	E/Air	Fixed	Acid	Gemi	Air	Mut	Alk	Mar incon merc	Red/lgt Brn/Silv	Massage head above ears
Jupiter	24° 59	Fire	Mut	Alk	4th	Water	Card	Acid	Leo	Fire	Fix	Alk	Vir Gem	Yellow/whit/Yell	
Saturn	25° 54R	Earth	Card	Acid	2nd	E/Air	Fixed	Acid	Gemi	Air	Mut	Alk	Saturns ruler ⚹ Gemini		Massage Celery Oil on Arms
Venus	27° 41	E/Air	F/Car	Alk/ac	5th	Fire	Fixed	Alk	Virgo	E/Air	M/M	Acid	Saturn □ Venus	Brown	
Neptune	03° 17	Water	Mut	Acid	5th	Fire	Fixed	Alk	Libra	Air	Card	Alk		Yellow/Pink	
MC	05° 21				10th				Aqua	Air	Fixed	Acid			
Uranus	07° 45R	Air	Fixed	Alk	2nd	E/Air	Fixed	Acid	Gemi	Air	Mut	Alk		P.Blue	Salt
Pluto	08° 45	Water	Fixed	Acid	4th	Water	Card	Acid	Leo	Fire	Fix	Alk	Pluto ruler □ Leo	Purple/Yellow	Potato with Oil for head

Chart 6

Inner Wheel N.R.
Natal Chart

Outer Wheel

7 Nov 1943
6:30 pm AEDT -11:00
Mudgee, NSW
32°S36' 149°E35'
Geocentric
Tropical
Equal
True Node

N.R.   Prog 1970
Sec.Prog. SA in Long (583)
15 Feb 1970
4:00 pm AEDT -11:00
Mudgee, NSW
32°S36' 149°E35'
Geocentric
Tropical
Equal
True Node

This chart shows the stroke patient Neville R.'s Natal Chart in the inner wheel and Progressed chart in the outer for the approximate period of when the stroke took place. I don't believe it requires a *flow chart* only that it would help to show in another form the planets degrees and their elements. It would be a formality to look at this if you wanted to know what could have affected him at the time the stroke took place, but it wouldn't be necessary for a formula.

In this chart the Sun, Mercury and Venus mightn't be accurately placed as it's going by memory of what the patient said several years earlier. But we could look at the outer planets and their progression and how they have affected the Natal chart.

When we look at a person who has had a illness and in this case a stroke we have to consider what has happened and what has been affected; Neville R. couldn't physically move his left arm or leg, in fact one would expect that his organs to some extent had been paralysed on the left side as well, but then again because the brain is ruled by Mercury and the legs are ruled by Jupiter maybe they are the two aspects we should be looking at. I did expect problems with the eye and mouth, but, he didn't appear to have the later problem. As mercury can't be ascertained as accurate in the progress chart we could look at the slower planets that were in Gemini the constellation ruled by Mercury, we couldn't guarantee the house so we can't look at the 3rd house.

Mercury still rules the arms which we can see in the Natal Chart as being 12° 04' Scorpio, Mercury in Scorpio already shows 150° if looked at in its natural sign of Gemini and so when met with other aspects is in a delicate position. The arms are an outer expression of the lungs in astrology and, if we look at Gemini the progress Mars has moved to 150° aspect to the Natal Sun and Mercury. Mars rules the red blood, head and muscles of the body. I would be concerned about exerting oneself in a physical manner, the Mars influence is hot and fiery, it is an active planet, but when in Gemini it's asking for it to be more talkative, an outcome of this would mean talking too fast, possibly burning up the oxygen. Natal Mercury is a degree earlier than the Mars degree so this is more likely to mean the gush of air would affect the muscles in the lungs, Mars ruler of muscles. Another quincunx 150° is Pluto to the Natal Moon. Pluto rules the groin and the hormones and its action is to be massive as

the oceans. It usually has a good affiliation to the Moon but when making this angle we could be concerned about too much moisture or too many polluted fluids flowing into the lymph nodes. Pluto squaring natal Mercury and it's own sign Scorpio would also bring about blockage to the Brain and Heart. According to the degrees it would first cause a problem with the brain ruled by Mercury which has a flow to the ☽ Moon being 19' later, which causes an already problematic area as earlier mentioned to Pluto. This is where the fluids could be too much. The Moon and Pisces are both water signs; Mercury in Scorpio is in a water sign. The Sun is in Scorpio and Pluto is squaring both Sun & Mercury. The Sun is the ruler of the heart and it shows that Mars was over-exerting the heart. With Mars 13° 36' and Sun 14° 01'.

The beauty of the North Node is that it is where the obvious focus is on. But, if they decide to look at an astrology chart and 150° aspects it is clear from a *flow chart* that we can look at a number of other areas.

The above chart shows how simply the problems of the heart can be corrected if they can take the emphasis away from death NN conjunct Pluto, Pluto is also remake or regeneration. From what I understand before the stroke he was a great sportsman.

The 29th March, 2003 was a milestone in discovery, it was the actual day we begun Neville R's. volunteered trials using the formulas made through what I could see in his chart, what was of great help was that he wanted to work on himself but more deeply his heart, Sun in Capricorn, 7th house meant in partnership. Mercury 21° 28'R in Capricorn in 8th House meant there would be deep research this was quincunx Saturn 21° 30'R Gemini on the 1st house cusp.

Chart 7

N.R. Progressed for

29 Mar 2003
10:00 am AEDT –11:00
Mudgee, NSW
32°S36' 149°E35'
Geocentric
Tropical
Equal
True Node

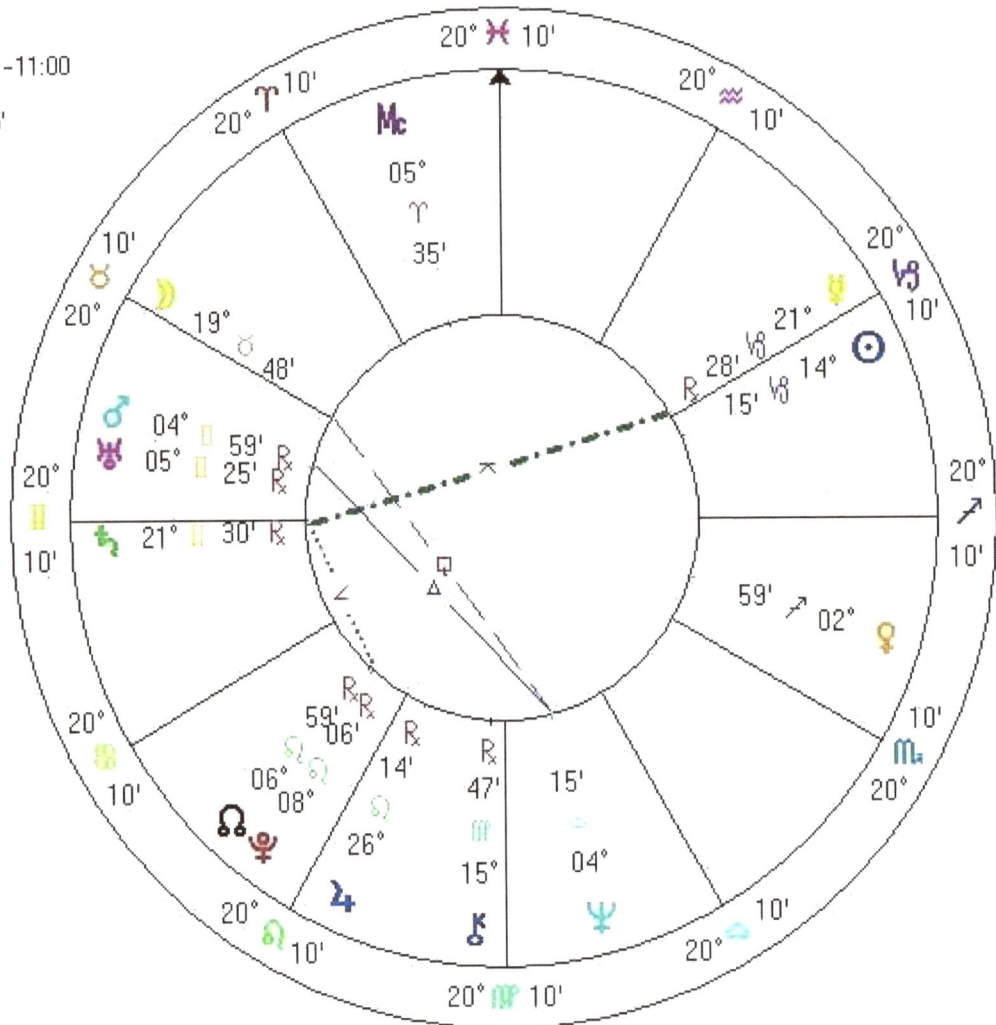

Whilst this was an area that needed to be looked at as it was a health aspect, 150°, individually it meant he was acceptable to his mind being changed. For 32 years he had never had any physiotherapy, and he admitted it to me that he just refused it at the time he left the hospital. They had told him he'd never walk and he did by his own recognizance, whilst struggling every step.

Neville R. had always enjoyed dancing, I had thought it was because of the stroke that when he did dance it was unpredictable and worrying. In looking at his chart when looking at the area that focuses on his legs we see Venus in Sagittarius, Sagittarius rules the Legs, this aspect is opposite to Mars one of the rulers of muscle conjuncting with 1° difference with Uranus one of the rulers of the circulation of the body it also rules the ankles, is the ruler of volcanos and unpredictable behaviour. When dancing it appeared that he wasn't conscious of fast and unpredictable movements. And, this would be natural with Mars and Uranus in the 12th House, which is ruled by Pisces, and probably why he could adapt to be crippled. The 12th house is said to show our own undoing; it's questionable whether this could be the case for Pisces or Neptune but there again it could mean depending on what planets are in it.

Now we'll look at Saturn 1st house, Sextile Jupiter ♃, Saturn shows the area he'd be working on, being in Gemini in the 1st house which is a cardinal or active house naturally shows he'd want to walk. This is a progressed sign and Saturn normally take 2 ½ years to go through a constellation

These works and records have been compiled over a period of 15 years. I'm not blessed with Jupiter in any favourable aspect except for freedom, and money certainly doesn't come easily for me; in some sense I was the silent partner in a marriage regarding finances, whilst I scrapped and saved for everything even when running a local paper nothing was easy, those problems came from often losing everything I wrote for an article and hadn't saved, I felt such an idiot. And when it came to everything I'd saved for it was all thrown away when a temporary separation took a more permanent arrangement and through illness I couldn't return. My husband saw no worth in anything I had created my Jupiter is in 8th house which has the characteristics of Scorpio being in a house position shows the area in which the action happens the actual constellation Jupiter is in, is that of Aries, which is direct active and straightforward; Partners are ruled by the 7th house with the characteristics of Libra. The Moon at 7° in Pisces is said to be a psychic sponge but at such time Pluto in Sagittarius was stronger for me not to know what was going on. Jupiter in Scorpio has given me the faith I have which I've mentioned earlier and that is the Magi Astrologer Priest often forgotten but were the followers of the star to Jesus ultimately the founders of Christianity; the Magi is believed to termed from the word 'magic' which appears now quiet irrelevant, astrology shows that some people have a gift of prophesy or the ability of illusion by a very swift hand, why I've gone into these areas I don't know all I do know is the depth in what I sometimes go coupled with my unpredictability, upsets my family and that which upsets the home upsets me. I know how and why it's caused and it would be with many people in my generation who have Uranus the feeling of unpredictability and freedom in the constellation of Cancer the home and family. Thou freedom without structure means you can lay down your roots in many places or not at all. My aspects are harsh *ones that oppose the brain (Mercury), the self (the Sun) and the intuition/psychic (Neptune) given that then I have a sextile from Pluto death destruction helps me to understand my life, to understand how things happen you do the flow chart which I've explained a number of times, based on degrees and minutes of the planets putting them in order from the Sun. I've been ever grateful for a man who was a guest speaker at Sydney Astrological Research Society, SARS teaching me that, I'm just sorry I can't remember his name.

Why have I waffled on, I guess it's to explain the 15 years in the making. When I began my research into the environment and not human nature, I desperately wanted a conclusive answer to whether was on the right path, whilst I believe there are many paths astrology can take us it is the degree in which part of physics you're at the lessor will only limit you to the heights you can go.

In 2006 early 2007 I sent most of my formulas to ANSTO they were based on carbons, to this date I haven't checked if any have been patented.

Inner Wheel
Wayne
Natal Chart (22)
1 Nov 1961
4:08 am AEST -10:00
Sydney, NSW
33'S52 151'E13'
Geocentric
Tropical
Placidus
True Node

Outer Wheel
Wayne
Sec.Prog. SA in Long (23)

4:08 am AEST -10:00
Sydney, NSW
33'S52 151'E13'
Geocentric
Tropical
Placidus
True Node

Chart 8

2007 was the same year I created a skin cancer formula for a gentleman I'll call by his first name Wayne, the heavens must have been with me. Of course when I first suggested I do a formula and there were his mates around they laughed. The problem is just as these men laughed at it people have lost the way of showing that by using what we have been told and have come true in the future it can go further. The initial question in my mind if God for another name gave us a predictive tool, a personality tool, why wouldn't he have given us a healing tool. My 2-year stint on 2BLU – Blue Mountains where I analysed current affairs issues and latest medical research showed to me God had. There was an acclaimed scientist who found mussels helped muscles and in Astrology by affiliation Aries/Mars/1st house rules muscles, to me it made sense that mussels could help muscles but it would have to be used in the correct way.

With the skin cancer formula, it was within days I had a formula, I was ecstatic, brain working/psychic working. I asked him to trial it and he said he would. The next time I saw him he had no sign of skin cancer I asked him to tell his doctor so that there would be some paper trail. I'd made a formula also up for his mate Dave S. I could take their sniggering because three of us were long term friends, Dave had suffered for a long time back pain and when he'd mentioned it before I thought it was temporary back pain, but when I took it seriously and made up a formula, he also came back and said it had worked.

These formulas may have only taken 56 hours to create but with my erratic emotional characteristic it was draining. And there again as what happened above happened again what I feel I've made from nothing was thrown away. For some reason they felt they couldn't defend keeping it, I presumed it wasn't their house. Strangely neither either of them ever had anything in their life, which was probably why they couldn't defend keeping them. It goes to show money isn't everything because at that time their support meant a great deal.

When looking at a chart you can also look at the situation surrounding people. Wayne was living with a family on a farm helping to raise wildlife and farm animals, but, I had felt and probably mentioned it to Wayne the philosophies of the family could possibly have caused the skin cancer, I say philosophies because Jupiter in astrology rules philosophies of others and in the anatomy the skin & liver. Where in health Jupiter was quincunx Uranus. But there's more which I'll go into when describing the formula's

In doing his mates chart who was nearly 40 and still lived with his parents, the astrological understanding to this is the back is said to have dual planets associated with it Saturn the bones, the Sun whilst it rules the heart it is closely associated with the spirit, but pride plays on structure. Figuratively it rules the Self, Son and the Father. I say the spirit because when I was told my mother had died. I sat with her and gradually followed her body going cold, and felt it was her spirit leaving her. It may have been the close Neptune association to the Sun, I'm not sure, in fact it's the first time I've mentioned it.

Getting back to the aspects, whilst there's a possibility the Sun has sort of a spiritual aspect, Saturn is the ruler of structure as I've often said, it's the builder, a negative aspect is deterioration of the bone structure, causing it to go crusty, medical term could have been arthritis but he never told me he had his back x-rayed. Externally, in Dave's case there was much pressure put on him by his Father and he was always called upon to move things or do things for his father, which would suddenly cause him to have to leave and go home. His father had been very active but, because he had his vertebrae fused he couldn't do things himself, and so in my analysis the external affected area had caused the internal reaction.

The same philosophy I'd use for a person dying of cancer, it's not the cancer that is killing them, but it still needs to be treated, even when consciously becoming aware of the situation. In talking of Cancer the Cancerian sign is one of concern and worry, it's an active sign, cardinal. It's also seen with the Moon and 4th house, and it's where we harbour memories. When the Moon transits the constellation it will tell us how we will emotionally react.

Referring back to Wayne's Natal Chart his Moon was in Leo, in the 3rd house but, because it is several years ago, I'm not sure if the time was right but the opposites/square and quincunx's will be right. And the formula I created worked. In my notes I put alternate foods and ways of preparing them.

Looking at the flow chart there is only 1° orb in the square between Moon to Mars. Moon in Leo meant his emotions are very proud, but the work environment could be dirty and grimy which would emotionally upset him, he had a square to working, this is not unusual many people go to work and hate but, there's an incentive for them to keep doing it. As to the field of work the chart shows the Moon makes a quincunx to Saturn so in any type of work he'd find his emotions interfering with his work, which could be the memories he has of his upbringing,

Below is his Flow Chart I've put in the house position but, as I've said I'm not confident. I couldn't get the same time that initially put planets into the houses. It's probably so simple I've just overlooked the art.

W.R. Natal chart Converted to a Flow Chart for 1 Nov 1961

PLANET	Degree	Trip	Quad	Acid/Alk	HOUSE	Trip	Quad	Acid/Alk	CONSTELLATION	Trip	Quad	Acid/Alk	ASPECTS	Food
Jupiter	6 52	Fire	Mutable	Alkaline	5th	Fire	Fixed	Acid	Aquarius	Air	Fixed	Alkaline	Jup□ Sn	Animal/
Sun	8 05	Fire	Fixed	Alkaline	6th	Earth	Mutable	Alkaline	Scorpio	Water	Fixed	Acid		Liver
Pluto	9 41	Water	Fixed	Acid	3rd	Air	Mutable	Acid	Virgo	Earth	Mutable	Acid		
Neptune	10 56	Water	Mutable	Acid	6th	Earth	Mutable	Alkaline	Scorpio	Water	Fixed	Acid	Nep □ Mn	Fish/
Moon	12 14	Water	Cardinal	Acid	11th	Air	Fixed	Alkaline	Leo	Fire	Fixed	Alkaline		pd milk/
*Neptune	12 30	Water	Mutable	Acid	6th	Earth	Mutable	Acid	Scorpio	Water	Fixed	Acid		Oranges
Venus	12 30	Earth/Air	Cardinal	Alk/Acid	2nd	Earth	Fixed	Acid	Sagittarius	Fire	Fixed	Alkaline		
Venus	16 55	Earth/Air	Fix/Card	Acid/Alk	5th	Fire	Fixed	Alkaline	Libra	Air	Cardinal	Alkaline		
11th Node	19 46R				11th	Air	Fixed	Alkaline	Leo	Fire	Fixed	Alkaline		
Mars	20 39	Fire	Cardinal	Alkaline	1st	Fire	Cardinal	Alkaline	Scorpio	Water	Fixed	Acid		Pepper
Mercury	22 10	Air/Earth	Mutable	Alk/Acid	3rd	Air	Mutable	Alkaline	Sagittarius	Fire	Mutable	Alkaline		
Mercury	22 19	Air/Earth	Card/Mut	Alk/Acid	1st	Fire	Cardinal	Alkaline	Libra	Air	Cardinal	Alkaline	Merc □ Sat	Celery
Mars	22 47	Fire	Cardinal	Alkaline	3rd	Air	Mutable	Alkaline	Sagittarius	Fire	Mutable	Alkaline		
Sun	22 52	Fire	Fixed	Alkaline	3rd	Air	Mutable	Alkaline	Sagittarius	Fire	Mutable	Alkaline		
Nth Node	24 11				11th	Air	Fixed	Alkaline	Leo	Fire	Fixed	Alkaline	NN ⚹ Sat	
Saturn	24 11	Earth	Cardinal	Acid	4th	Water	Cardinal	Acid	Capricorn	Earth	Cardinal	Acid	Leo ⚹ Cap	Oil
Moon	26 10	Water	Cardinal	Acid	6th	Earth	Mutable	Acid	Pisces	Water	Mutable	Acid		
Saturn	27 49	Earth	Cardinal	Acid	4th	Water	Cardinal	Acid	Capricorn	Earth	Cardinal	Acid		
Jupiter	29 06	Fire	Mutable	Alkaline	4th	Water	Cardinal	Acid	Capricorn	Earth	Cardinal	Acid	Jup ⚹ Ur	Liver
Uranus	29 58	Air	Fixed	Alkaline	11th	Air	Fixed	Alkaline	Virgo	Earth	Mutable	Acid	Ur □ Chir	Salt
Uranus	00 31R	Air	Fixed	Alkaline	11th	Air	Fixed	Alkaline	Virgo	Earth	Mutable	Acid		
Chiron	01 57	Not Enough Information			9th	Fire	Mutable	Alkaline	Pisces	Water	Mutable	Acid		

Green is the progressed planets

With Wayne I took a different approach to other formulas. I could clearly see the skin cancer and so I focused on his arms; immediately looking in his chart for Mercury/Jupiter and Saturn/Capricorn aspects; and, of course Pluto. As you can see Pluto is only 1 degree from the Sun. The aspects to constellations is not harsh. But, there is a 210 deg made between Aquarius & Virgo the alternate partner to a quincunx.

Progressed Jupiter is in Aquarius squaring Sun and Pluto; Mercury square Saturn; Natal Jupiter quincunx's Uranus

In focusing on these aspects we see: -

Progressed Jupiter in Aquarius Square Sun in Scorpio

This means he'd have problems with weight/problems with liver. It means his hopes probably would have been adverse to his fathers. It indicates to combine in the formula- air dried liver with Oranges and salt

Mercury in Libra Square Saturn in Capricorn
Mercury has to do with arms, breathing, brain, the nervous system and air, being in Libra means there would be a doubling of air and a sweetness; being square means the air would be blocked by the influence of Saturn, and there would be breathing problems. Asthma/Emphysema, his breathing was stressed at the time I wasn't focusing on lung illnesses, but of course it was indicated with skin cancer on the arms, without realising it when doing formulas, you can be helping other problem. But, Saturn in Capricorn gives a double influence. Capricorn/Saturn element earth has a gravely/soil effect.

Saturn is 5 degrees away from Jupiter, this means he'd be quite joyful when working, but almost immediately he gets started he'd be called away, with the Uranus 150 deg. aspect, this wouldn't be good for permanent work. With Saturn we get a crust when aspects affect it. Saturn with Jupiter would normally be productive, but Uranus which rules wild animals up until 2 months earlier he'd been helping to look after wildlife at home. it's made a health aspect

What I'm going to do unlike previous explanations I'm going to write the formula and show the influence.

Formula
Cow Liver to charcoal
Olive Oil
Salt
Water
Orange Juice
Previous made Pepper Celery cooked and dried
Hoki dried

I've omitted quantities because they change and are individual.

Capricorn also refers to coal/charcoal
Oranges are excellent for Magnesium a product required for the heart and the Sun is round and Orange.
Liver is a product of Jupiter for skin, I possibly could have used chicken livers they would have combined both Mercury and Jupiter and cause the formula to have more coverage.
Salt is a product of Uranus

When Jupiter is in Capricorn we are looking for something that renews itself or expands, we never think of the skin renewing itself but if we have a cut it eventually sows itself up in a healthy person. We often hear of the liver growing when parts have been cut off, these are the two functioning rulerships of Jupiter. Jupiter being in Capricorn means we want something that will eventually form a structure or is active, its element is earth Jupiter's the planet that rules philosophies/religions and law. An obvious food group of Jupiter is by now shouldn't be surprising

71

is liver which can be bought in any supermarket I was torn between 3 food groups liver/ bacon chips & pork, I used liver because, I've never found it to fail, another quality I was looking for was earth substance required by Capricorn and earth is created by the drying substances, and because Jupiter has a fire element, this led me to put the liver under the grill to dry it out. The next step was to find not the element of Capricorn, but a material that had been doubly processed, oil has been contributed to Capricorn. The theory behind it is that as the earth ages it creates oil so to the formula I add 1/4 cup of Olive Oil with also a characteristic of Jupiter where a little bit goes a long way.

Where Mars is concerned there was a formula I had fallen back onto which I had made and used earlier. It was simple and affective I put pepper with celery and dried the ingredients in the microwave. Celery is an air product which is Gemini, I probably would have preferred comfrey but it's very hard to find and for myself harder to grow, why because the description of the buds of the comfrey plant are described as a hand usually having 5 flowers and the skin cancer affected his hands and arms. The Asians believe it has many beneficial qualities, and I've read so has celery but not as much potassium, in saying that it has a high degree of sodium mixing it with pepper added the potassium where combined gives a Mars/Mercury influence, whilst there is little carbohydrates in celery I've read and interestingly on the internet under 'what is celery high in' that the calories in the celery comes from sugars, but, the good qualities far outweigh the bad. But, there again in using celery it added the natural sugars I required for Mercury being in Libra.

The Moon and Neptune square led me to add Hoki they feed on small crustaceans which is ruled by Saturn it's found in the oceans which is ruled by Scorpio/Pluto which relates to the Neptunian and Sun influence we see in Scorpio. The process I took was to cook it in a little bit of water let it dry out and combined the below ingredient to rub into his chest and ankles.

Over 15 years I've worked on many areas the above have been the more intense. Before I go on I should mention that my own health history has constantly changed which I mentioned in the early part of this book, when I've concentrated on my own health I've seemed to have problem areas disappear i.e. diabetes which didn't show up in my last blood test which has amazed doctors, on rare occasions I'd inform them that I was working on my own health formulas. The following outline those minor areas I've worked on for the many people who have passed through my life :-

Acute Anaemia; Continual headaches; Back pain; Pain through back fusion; Smokers cough; Vaginal itching; Hives; Sore throat; Boils; Broken toe pain; a neighbour who had bone cancer and a reaction to tablets, when his family thought he was looking better they took him away; Goiter; Leukemia with friend; Severe neck pain.

Inner Wheel
David S.
Natal Chart (27)
2 Oct 1973
3:00 am AEST -10:00
Sydney, NSW
33°S52' 151°E13'
Geocentric
Tropical
Placidus
True Node

Outer Wheel
David S.
Sec.Prog. SA in Long (28)
3 Mar 2007
12:01 pm AEST -10:00
Sydney, NSW
33°S52' 151°E13'
Geocentric
Tropical
Placidus
True Node

Chart 9

Above is David's Natal Chart (Inner Wheel) and Progressed Chart (Outer Wheel). Chart 10 shows the aspects he was born with, the red line show considerable squares, whilst he had the ability to overlook them with a cheerful outer appearance when with others, and there was an easy flow with his family, as long as he didn't work. It also shows that he was in tune mentally with his father, but physically not able to cope and that the father would put the pressure on him with Saturn being prior to the Sun which is the physical being. There was an obvious opposition with Uranus Mars and Mercury and for some reason going through my notes I didn't put it in but, I did add a transiting aspect of Uranus in Pisces. And in the formula there is a food for Mars which is pepper and Mercury which is celery.

73

David S.
Natal Chart (27)
2 Oct 1973
3:00 am AEST -10:00
Sydney, NSW
33°S52' 151°E 13'
Geocentric
Tropical
Placidus
True Node

Chart 10

Pain is evident with Saturn Square Pluto and the Sun. There is also Mars making 150 deg. Angle to the Sun.

Below is David's Flow Chart putting planets in order of degrees helps to know which order one prepares the food. When there are conjuncts you combine; aspects up to 10 deg. away you prepare separately; sometimes I've done 3 separate formulas, with N.R. I was preparing formulas on the spot in particular making massage oils apart from acupuncture and hypnosis.

The foods I chose were those in the flow chart, the final product was rubbed into his back. I've noticed the Uranus influence missing were I did add Mushrooms this carries water and unpredictably grows in moist weather.

The foods I used took into consideration the Planet House and Constellation e.g. Jupiter/Liver, Saturn/Mylanta, Cancer/Milk, Neptune Wine. In my notes I haven't put the exact time which makes the house positions dubious. Whilst the formula worked, on what I did, but obviously I would have had the correct time.

D.S. Natal & Progressed Flow Chart based on DOB & 3 March 2007

PLANET	Degree	Trip	Quad	Acid/Alk	HOUSE	Trip	Quad	Acid/Alk	CONSTELLATION	Trip	Quad	Acid/Alk	ASPECTS	Food
Jupiter	2 18	Fire	Mutable	Alk	6th	Earth	Mutable	Acid	Aquarius	Air	Fixed	Alk	Jup/Sat	Cow Liver
Jupiter	4 25	Fire	Mutable	Alk	6th	Earth	Mutable	Acid	Aquarius	Air	Fixed	Alk	Jup/Sun	Mylanta
Pluto‡	4 27	Water	Fixed	Acid	2nd	Earth	Fixed	Acid	Libra	Air	Cardinal	Alk		Pd Milk
Saturn	4 27 R	Earth	Cardinal	Acid	11th	Air	Fixed	Alk	Cancer	Water	Cardinal	Acid		Wine + Oil
Saturn	4 32	Earth	Cardinal	Acid	11th	Air	Fixed	Alk	Cancer	Water	Cardinal	Acid	Sat/Nep	Egg Shell
Neptune‡	5 14	Water	Mutable	Acid	4th	Water	Cardinal	Acid	Sagittarius	Fire	Mutable	Alk		Kelp
Pluto‡	5 39	Water	Fixed	Acid	2nd	Earth	Fixed	Acid	Libra	Air	Cardinal	Alk		Red Fish
Mars	8 15 R	Fire	Cardinal	Alk	9th	Fire	Mutable	Alk	Taurus	Earth	Fixed	Acid	Mar/Sun	Cow Necks
Sun	8 22	Fire	Fixed	Alk	2nd	Earth	Fixed	Acid	Libra	Air	Cardinal	Alk		Pepper Grain
Moon	8 41	Water	Cardinal	Acid	4th	Water	Cardinal	Acid	Sagittarius	Fire	Mutable	Alk		Oranges
Sun	11 33	Fire	Fixed	Alk	3rd	Air	Mutable	Alk	Scorpio	Water	Fixed	Acid	Sun/Mn	
Chiron	17 36	Insufficient Information			8th	Water	Fixed	Acid	Aries	Fire	Cardinal	Alk		
Moon	21 03	Water	Cardinal	Acid	6th	Earth	Mutable	Acid	Aquarius	Air	Fixed	Alk	Mn/Vn	
Venus	21 17	E/Air	Fix/Card	Acid/Alk	3rd	Air	Mutable	Alk	Scorpio	Water	Fixed	Acid		
Uranus‡	22/24	Air	Fixed	Alk	2nd	Earth	Fixed	Acid	Libra	Air	Cardinal	Alk		
Mercury	24 57	Air/Earth	Mutable	Acid/Alk	3rd	Air	Mutable	Alk	Scorpio	Water	Fixed	Acid		
Mercury	28 23	Air/Earth	Mutable	Acid/Alk	2nd	Earth	Fixed	Acid	Libra	Air	Cardinal	Alk	Merc/NN	Celery
Venus	28 24	E/Air	Fix/Card	Acid/Alk	5th	Fire	Fixed	Alk	Sagittarius	Fire	Mutable	Alk		
Nth Node	29 47	Air/Earth	Mutable	Alk	5th	Fire	Fixed	Alk	Sagittarius	Fire	Mutable	Alk		Cod Liver
Nth Node	2 22	E/Air	Fix/Card	Acid	5th	Fire	Fixed	Alk	Capricorn	Earth	Cardinal	Acid		Oil

Chart 11

Inner Wheel
N.S.
Natal Chart (29)
8 Jan 1970
9:30 am AEST -10:00
Sydney, NSW
33°S52' 151°E13'
Geocentric
Tropical
Placidus
True Node

Outer Wheel
N.S.
Sec.Prog. SA in Long (30)
20 Apr 2016
9:05 pm AEST -10:00
Sydney, NSW
33°S52' 151°E13'
Geocentric
Tropical
Placidus
True Node

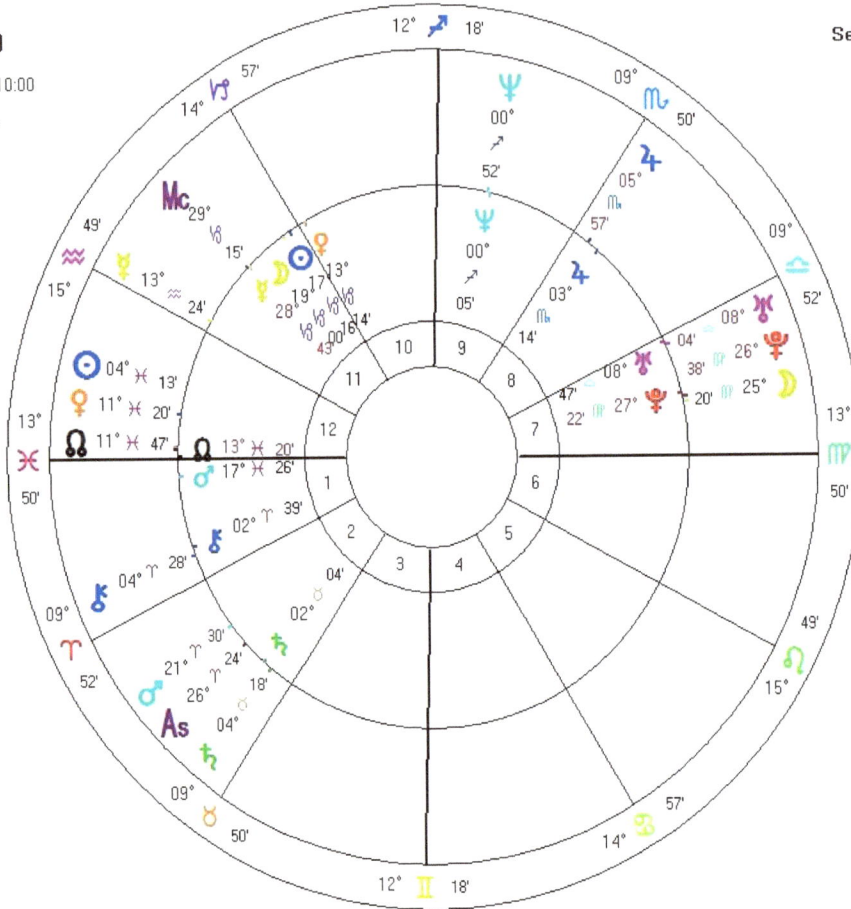

V.S. Natal & Progressed Flow Chart based on DOB & 20 April 2016

PLANET	Degree	Trip	Quad	Alk/Acid	HOUSE	Trip	Quad	Alk/Acid	CONSTELLATION	Trip	Quad	Alk/Acid	Aspect	Food
Sun	04 13	Fire	Fixed	Alk	11th	Air	Fixed	Alk	Pisces	Water	Mutable	Acid	Pl/Sun	Calc Sulph
Saturn	04 18	Earth	Cardinal	Acid	2nd	Earth	Fixed	Acid	Taurus	Earth	Fixed	Acid		& Magnesium
Chiron	04 28				1st	Fire	Cardinal	Alk	Aries	Fire	Cardinal	Alk		
Jupiter	05 57	Fire	Mutable	Alk	8th	Water	Fixed	Acid	Scorpio	Water	Fixed	Acid		
Uranus	08 04 R	Air	Fixed	Alk	7th	Air	Cardinal	Alk	Libra	Air	Cardinal	Alk	Sun/Ur	
Uranus*	08 47	Air	Fixed	Alk	7th	Air	Cardinal	Alk	Libra	Air	Cardinal	Alk	Ur/Venus	Salt/Sugar
Venus	11 20	Ea/Air	Fix/Card	Ac/Alk	12th	Water	Mutable	Acid	Pisces	Water	Mutable	Acid		
Nth Node*	11/13 deg	Ea/Air	Fix/Card	Ac/Alk	12th	Water	Mutable	Acid	Pisces	Water	Mutable	Acid		
Venus	13 14	Ea/Air	Fix/Card	Ac/Alk	10th	Earth	Cardinal	Acid	Capricorn	Earth	Cardinal	Acid		
Mercury	13 24	Air/Ea	Mut/Mut	Alk/Acid	11th	Air	Fixed	Alk	Aquarius	Air	Fixed	Alk		
Sun	17 16	Fire	Fixed	Alk	11th	Air	Fixed	Alk	Capricorn	Earth	Cardinal	Acid	Sun/Mars	
Mars	17 26	Fire	Cardinal	Alk	1st	Fire	Cardinal	Alk	Pisces	Water	Mutable	Acid		pd milk/water
Moon	19 00	Water	Cardinal	Acid	11th	Air	Fixed	Alk	Capricorn	Earth	Cardinal	Acid	Mn/Mars	Chilli sauce
Mars	21 30	Fire	Cardinal	Alk	2nd	Earth	Fixed	Acid	Aries	Fire	Cardinal	Alk	Mars/Mn	Orange Pepper
Moon	25 20	Water	Cardinal	Acid	7th	Air	Cardinal	Alk	Virgo	Earth	Mutable	Acid		
Pluto*	26/27 deg	Water	Fixed	Acid	7th	Air	Cardinal	Alk	Virgo	Earth	Mutable	Acid	Pl/Nept	Fermented
Mercury	28 43	Air/Ea	Mut/Mut	Alk/Acid	11th	Air	Fixed	Alk	Capricorn	Earth	Cardinal	Acid		Hoki & Kelp
Neptune	00 05/52'	Water	Mutable	Acid	8th	Water	Fixed	Acid	Sagittarius	Fire	Mutable	Alk	Nept/Sat	Grilled Liver
Saturn	02 04	Earth	Cardinal	Acid	2nd	Earth	Fixed	Acid	Taurus	Earth	Fixed	Acid	Sat/Jup	Gin-Charcoal
Jupiter	03 14	Fire	Mutable	Alk	8th	Water	Fixed	Acid	Scorpio	Water	Fixed	Acid		Horse Fertsiliser

SEVERE PERIOD PAIN

Above, with the first Astrology Chart I have combined the natal and progress planetary aspects for Nicky S for this current time, it is a sudden impulse to include her chart because there is a lot to learn from it, I feel. Nicky and I, became friends just over 10 years ago and whilst I've given her a formula I'd created, I found she kept using something the Doctor would give her to trial and for a long while they never reached the desired goal or they were just too expensive to buy. I was actually living in Parkes at the time we met and I had opened shop so to speak, but I've found working for myself is just untimely as my chart shows, so having my mind on creating a full formula was too stressful. You're always looking for the dollar when you work for yourself. And whilst I had included Astrology I was looking into law and legal forms for the public.

Nicky and I only knew each other for about 6 months when periodically she had what appeared to be menstrual problems. Menstrual problems for women are just natural; and one expects discomfort; but, change of life at 36 is a bit early.

I'd remember she told me that she was waking up in cold sweats drenched. Which I believe has continues till this day

I remember starting a few times to do a formula for her, but I wasn't in the right mind space. This is important, whilst a flippant remark, the mind is ruled by Mercury and Mercury rules Gemini and Virgo. As a consequence, I said to her 'I mightn't be able to do a formula for you'. In what I said I realise now, it all had to do with timing, and in reflecting in her progressed chart for 2006. I can clearly see now my natal Nth Node is conjuncting her Nth Node in Pisces with a 4° difference. And being opposite to Virgo means opposite to formulas. Pisces has to do with instinct and alcohol, and there were many a memorable time. But it is opposite to being practical and looking into health issues. As such my comment was instinctual and, correct.

Later in 2011 when I lived down in Wollongong I tried again this time I was able to do a partial formula, where she informed me it worked, but she had discontinued using it because when the symptoms came on, it was in the middle of the night and she couldn't bring herself to rub a fine granule formula on herself. I remember it had to do with seaweed. And, looking at the progressed chart for 2006 below it shows North Node, Sun and Venus in Pisces 12th house relating intensively to sleep. This means she could have been suffering from anaemia and a lazy thyroid; and, if I remember correctly she did tell me doctors thought there were thyroid problems.

I found out recently that she'd been sick for the last 2 weeks with serious back pain with extremely heavy period, and for many years she hadn't slept in her own bed. This time I've found my mind is not so subjective meaning full of personal feeling, BECAUSE I realize we didn't only have our Nth Nodes conjunct, my moon is also conjuncting the Nth Nodes, which makes an easy flow to Jupiter in Aries in 8th house (8th house is everything or nothing). Which is opposite my Natal Saturn. And, I've found work brings no joy. It reminds me of how it used to upset my daughter in particular when I worked from home, and this is an obvious outcome with Saturn making a 150° to Moon & North Node.

With Nicky's chart going purely by the symptoms you'd expect to see the planet that gives pain, Saturn involved, (write these down) Saturn also rules the vertebrae of the body. For the pain to be so severe for having to take 2 weeks off work, it meant something would have emphasised it. When we look at direct oppositions we see Saturn conjunct Saturn in Taurus, Taurus is also the ruler of the 2nd house where these two planets are, as such we have two planets in Taurus both in the 2nd house which gives an emphasis of 4. This causes gravel, being opposite the natal and progressed Jupiter that rules the Liver means Saturn would be stopping the necessary hormone for the liver to function properly, thyroxine. This is because Thyroid is ruled by Taurus. This. aspect would also cause a problem with her periods because of Saturn in Taurus.

Natal and Progressed Jupiter are both in Scorpio, Scorpio rules the Reproductive Organs and Jupiter rules excess. Jupiter is the planet that rules Sagittarius which are known for their extravagance and would be the cause of the heavy and excessive bleeding. When Jupiter is in Scorpio, and 8th house, normally ruled by Scorpio – I'd be confident in using the oil from horse manure, Sagittarius symbol being the Centaur half man half horse, 8th house rules manure. Of course I wouldn't include it without permission, and when I first used it with Wayne, he praised me immediately, this came after other formulas and had an instant effect on allowing him to breath. Where in truth I needed to do extra formulas on other planetary aspects I neglected. Returning to Nicky, it shows that Jupiter makes a positive aspect to the Sun if Saturn hadn't been causing so much pain.

Aspects of Nicky haven't moved much in 10 years and can be seen in both charts 14 and 15, one has to realise that the planets for a progressed chart will have only moved 46 days. (Refer Planets Movements for more information). In saying that the Moon has moved the furthest, where it was in Taurus and now in Virgo.

When North Node is in Pisces it also accompanies fear. Fear that things can't be done. It makes things either very confused or very spiritual. Because Nicky and I had formed a deep bond it made me fearful that I'd miss something and fail. With Nicky's North Nodes they give he the ability of perception because of the natural flow to the Sun and a number of planets. She has a beauty which is noticed with Venus conjunct. But, she often says to people who compliment her that it's not external beauty that counts. This straight forwardness comes from the Moon square Mars, where there is a double Mars influence with Mars in Aries, in 2006 Mars directness flowed on to the male form, where it has moved on where she might get abused by males, working in an aged care centre. In addition, the North Node and Venus are in Pisces, this means she wouldn't see herself as others do, but it's also accompanied by her Natal Mercury is in Capricorn which brings about focus.

Where I first mentioned Nicky having Night sweats and waking up soaking wet the first thing the Doctors thought was that it related to menopause, a time when a woman has irregular periods and where the blood flow can be erratic. But, in fact night sweats relate to the planet Mars and constellation Aries. When it was first happening Natal Mars is in Pisces in its own 1st house. This would mean excessive sweating whilst asleep when Mars is affected. But it becomes more obvious with Progressed Mars squaring the Sun. Mars rules the 'red' blood cells. In the flow chart I've suggested Orange Peppers.

Unfortunately, I haven't the facility to make the formula up, and these aspects for some are constant because of the progressed planets, or because of the persons own natal chart, but what influenced the illness were the transiting planets, where her illness lasted a fortnight. Progressed signs can take 4 to 5 years to get over, and if there is another planet close another type of illness will show up. I haven't done enough research to know how long my formulas work only for Neville who had a stroke, and returned to limping after 15 months when his doctor couldn't get rid of a lump in his good leg.

Because I've omitted the Transits, I've included chart 16 for the 5 April 2016. Where the red lines show the number of planets affecting us at that time. The other unfortunate thing for myself is that Astrology is discriminated against and if a patient is unwilling to trial the formula, it would be necessary to talk to a doctor with an open mind and to get over prejudices, and this illusion that god didn't give us a path.

I've given the foods in the Flow Chart and the preparation is in the elements. The symbol of Constellations has already given us the primary food to work from. Whilst not required in Nicky's chart, with Gemini and Libra I use the anatomy part it rules i.e. sheep/cow brains; for Libra is cow's Kidney.

Alternatives are given under Foods of Constellations, for Libra problems relating to Kidneys, lately and I feel so stupid in saying this, I've found bi-carbonated soda should be looked into for those on dialysis, but in very small amounts in water. Soda is a cell salt for Libra and its planet Venus has 96.5% Carbon Dioxide, and in giving it to a father whose young child was in hospital for kidney problems, she was out in a few days instead of the weeks they thought she'd be in there.

Chart 12

Inner Wheel
N.S.
Natal Chart (29)
8 Jan 1970
9:30 am AEST −10:00
Sydney, NSW
33°S52' 151°E13'
Geocentric
Tropical
Placidus
True Node

Outer Wheel
N.S.
Sec.Prog. SA in Long (31)
10 May 2006
9:05 pm AEST −10:00
Sydney, NSW
33°S52' 151°E13'
Geocentric
Tropical
Placidus
True Node

Chapter 12 - Calculating Your Chart Manually

The following works of Ursula Lewis who wrote 'Chart our Own Horoscope', is one of the best examples I've ever come across giving full examples which you can understand by following the steps which are outlined in text as well as providing illustrations   You'll find it handy if you wish to sit the American or Australian Federation of Astrologer's FAA exam . Though it's not in its entirety the later part of this chapter gives the calculations for understanding the planets movements. I am putting this first because if you're at all sceptical you'll realise you'll need brains as well as beauty to go on. Except for those who've got computers :)

Text books required are: -

1. A Table of Houses

2. A book on Longitude and Latitude of the World

3. The Prime Meridians

4. A book showing Time Changes

5. Ephemeris giving sidereal time and planetary positions for a given date.

6. Table of proportional logarithms you will require in particular Table 33, Appendix A

7. A blank birth chart.

To calculate a chart, we begin with Date of Birth, Time of Birth and Place of Birth, it doesn't need to be a person it could be a country or event and we continue as follows:

Abbrev: L.M.T. > Local Mean Time; E.G.M.T. > Equivalent Greenwich Mean Time; ST. T. > Standard Time

Date: 7 November, 1972. Time: 2:24 pm ST.T. (Standard Time). Place: Los Angeles, Ca.

Longitude	Latitude	L.M.T	E.G.M.T.
118° W15'	34° N03'	+7m 00s	+7h 53m 00s

(For conversion for Longitude refer The Prime Meridians)
(E.G.M.T. found in the Ephemeris)
Steps:

	Hours	Minutes	Seconds
1. Clock time at p.m. birth	02	24	00 ST. T.
2. Local Mean Time is a variation from birth time and gives >	+	7	00

	Hour	Minute	Seconds
True Local Time =	02	31	00
3. 10 Second Interval Correction	+		26
This is a calculation on hr & mins 1 Hr = 10s 1-6 min = 1s	02	31	26
4. Sidereal Time of the 7th as birth occurred after 12 Noon	+15	07	08
	17	38	34
5. Longitudinal Correction (Formula: Multiply by 2, divide result by 3, Always Add result when birth place was west of Greenwich; deduct result when birth place is east of Greenwich)	+00	01	19
The final calculated Sidereal Time = 17		39	53

Brought Forward	Hour	Minute	Seconds
The final calculated Sidereal Time =	17	39	53

This figure is used in the Table of Houses along with the Latitude to find the Ascendant, Medium Coeli M.C., Nadir, Descendent & other 8 house positions.

6. Refer Step 2 the True Local

		Hour	Minute	Seconds
Time	02	31	00	
Refer E.G.M.T.	+07	53	00	
	09	94		00

The 6th Step is used to find planetary movements by converting the h/m/s into a logarithm the 9h 94m Equivalent = 10hrs 24m 00s
This is the Greenwich Mean Time on the 7th Nov.

The C.L. (Constant Log) for 10hr 24m = .3632 (This is the planetary correction between 7th and 8th November)

Equations

The earth is divided into twenty-four prime meridians, each one 15° distant from the next. This is longitude calculation. From Greenwich Observatory in England, which has been designated as 0°. (See The Prime Meridian Table). In all places clocks are synchronized to the standard time in that prime meridian. This system has the obvious advantage of standardization, but it does not assure true time. Unless a person was born exactly on a prime meridian, the true time of his birth is not the same as the official time. Hence the official time has to be converted to True Local Time.

To return to our example: The clocks for Los Angeles are set for the 120th prime meridian, but since Los Angeles is only 118° N15' it is actually 1° 45' east of its prime meridian or true time centre. Now, the Sun travels 1° every 4 minutes, and 15° x 4 minutes equals 60 minutes, which equals 1 hour. This is why each of the prime meridians are 15° for 1 hour apart. Since Los Angeles is short by 1° 45' of the nearest prime meridian, and 1° is equivalent to 4 minutes of the time and 45' is equivalent to 3 minutes of time, the difference between the True Local Time and the official time is Los Angeles is 7 minutes. The 7 minutes are added to the official time. The 7 minutes are added to the official time because Los Angeles is east of its true time centre. (If the birthplace is west of the prime meridian, then the time difference is subtracted.)

In the Birth Calculation, Step 1 the clock time is noted as 2 hours, 24 minutes, 00 seconds. Since Daylight Saving Time was not in effect in November 1972 it is Marked ST. T. which stands for Standard Time. At this point let me note that we are working with a *noontime ephemeris* in which each day begins at Greenwich Noon Time and ends at noon the next day. From 12 Noon 7 November 1972, 2 hours, 24 minutes and 00 seconds have passed in our example case.

Step 2 concerns the Local Mean Time variation in this case the adjustment is 7 minutes, 00 seconds, and it is added to the clock time.
Step 3 is a 10-second interval correction. Here we begin to adjust for Sidereal Time. *Sidereal Time progresses by approximately 4 minutes per day.*

The 4 minutes-per-day accumulation time 4 years equals just slightly over 24 hours, or one extra day – which is inserted into our calendar in February 29 every four years. Sidereal Time is the most accurate method of time reckoning and is used in every astronomical observatory.

Since the ephemeris gives only one Sidereal Time per day –with all ephemeris usually an adjustment has to be made if the birth time was not exactly noon or midnight, in this case noon. The calculations in the

above example has a correction of 26 seconds, which is obtained from **The Prime Meridians**, which I included for your convenience. By checking the Prime Meridians, you will note that Two hours require a correction of 20 seconds, and 31 minutes require a correction of 6 seconds. The 10-second interval correction of 26 seconds is added to the L.M.T of 2 hours, 31 minutes, 00 seconds for a total of 2 hours, 31 minutes, 26 seconds (Step 1 plus 2, plus 3).

For **Step 4** we have to consult *Raphael's Ephemeris*, November 1972. The ephemeris page for 7 November shows the Sidereal Time as 15 hours, 07 minutes 08 seconds. We add this Sidereal Time to Step 3, which gives a total of 17 hours, 38 Minutes, 34 seconds.

Step 5 is the *longitudinal correction*. The rule for this is s follows. Longitude times 2 divided by 3. The longitude of Los Angeles is 118° W15' . Multiply 118 by 2, which gives 236. Divide this figure by 3 and the result is 78 with 2 remaining. Since the remainder is more than half the divisor, the total is rounded off to 79. This correction is always in seconds; 79 seconds would be 1 minute and 19 seconds. The longitudinal correction is *added to the Sidereal Time:* the result in the Calculations above is 17 hours, 39 minutes, 53 seconds – the Final Calculated True Local Sidereal Time.

Notice that we dropped the 15' in the 118° W 15' longitude figure. Whenever the minute figure is less than 30, it is dropped. If it is more than 30, the degree figure is increased by 1. Also note that the longitudinal correction is *added if the birthplace was west* of Greenwich but *deducted if the birthplace was east* of Greenwich. With the completion of Step 5, we are ready to set up the horoscope wheel.

TABLE OF HOUSES

TABLE OF HOUSES FOR LATITUDES 20° to 56°

UPPER MERIDIAN, CUSP OF 10th H.

	H.	M.	S.			H.	M.	S.			H.	M.	S.
SID. T.	17	33	51}	♐		17	38	13}	♐ 25°		17	42	34}
ARC	263° 27'.8		} 24°			264° 33'.1 }					265° 38.5'}		

Lat.	11 ♑	12 ♒	1 ♓	2 ♈	3 ♉	11 ♑	12 ♒	1 ♓	2 ♈	3 ♓	11 ♑	12 ♒	1 ♓
22	18	16.6	21 23	28.5	29	19.8	18	22.5	29.8	30	21	19	24 15
23	19	16.3	21 17	28.7	29	19.6	18	22 44	29.9	30	21	18.8	24 11
24	18	16.1	21 11	28.9	29	19.5	17	22 39	0.1 ♉	30	21	18.5	24 07
25	18	15.8	21 5	29.1	29	19.3	17	22 34	0.3	♊	20	18.3	24 03
26	18	15.5	20 59	29.3	29	19.2	17	22 29	0.5	0.2	20	0	23 59
27	18	15.3	20 53	29.5	29	0	17	22 24	0.7	0.3	0	17.8	23 55
28	18	0	20 46	29.7	29	18.8	16	22 18	1	0.5	20	17.5	23 50
29	18	14.7	20 39	29.9	30	18.7	16	22 12	1.2	0.7	20	17.2	23 45
30	17	14.4	20 31	0.1 ♉	30	18.5	16	22 06	1.4	0.8	20	16.9	23 40
31	17	14.1	20 24	0.3	30	18.3	15	21 59	1.6	1	19	16.6	23 35
32	17	13.8	20 16	0.5	.0 ♊	18.1	0	21 52	1.9	1.2	19	16.3	23 29
33	17	13.4	20 7	0.8	0.3	17.9	15	21 45	2.1	1.4	0	0	23 23
34	17	13.1	19 58	1	0.5	17.7	14	21 38	2.4	1.5	19	15.6	23 17
35	17	12.7	19 48	1.3	0.7	17.5	0	21 30	2.7	1.7	19	15.3	23 11
36	16	12.3	19 38	1.6	0.9	17.3	14	21 21	3	1.9	18	14.9	23 04
37	0	11.9	19 27	1.9	1.1	17.1	13	21 12	3.3	2.1	18	14.5	22 57
38	16	11.5	19 16	2.2	1.3	16	13	21 02	3.6	2.4	18	14.1	22 49

Step 2

Table 1

The Prime Meridians

Meridian	Hrs East of Greenwich
180°	-12 (dateline)
165°	-11
150°	-10
135°	-9
120°	-8
105°	-7
90°	-6
75°	-5
60°	-4
45°	-3
30°	-2
15°	-1

0° Greenwich England. Observatory	
	Hrs West of Greenwich
15°	+1
30°	+2
45°	+3
60°	+4
75°	+5
90°	+6
105°	+7
120°	+8
135°	+9
150+	+9
150°	+10
165°	+11
180°	+12 Dateline

Step 3
10 Second Interval Correction

hr	hr	min	sec
1	00	00	10
2	00	00	20
3	00	00	30
4	00	00	40
5	00	00	50
6	00	01	00
7	00	01	10
8	00	01	20
9	00	01	30
10	00	01	40
11	00	01	50
12	00	02	00
13	00	02	10
14	00	02	20
15	00	02	30
16	00	02	40
17	00	02	50
18	00	03	00
19	00	03	10
20	00	03	20
21	00	03	30
22	00	03	40
23	00	03	50
24	00	04	0
Minute	**H**	**M**	**S**
1-6	00	00	01
7-12	00	00	02
13-18	00	00	03
19-24	00	00	04
25-30	00	00	05
31-36	00	00	06
37-42	00	00	07
43-48	00	00	08
49-54	00	00	09
55-60	00	00	10

House Cusps

The House cusps are found by referring to the Table of Houses. In the calculations first applied in the 5th Step it shows the final calculation performed for the Sidereal Time which came to 17hrs 39m 53s all else under it doesn't apply to this.   With this information we go to the Table of Houses which show the Latitude in the illustration we go to the page with Latitude that shows 22° to 56° the Latitude of Los Angeles is 34° N 03' in the Table it show the Sidereal Time closest to this, when you follow the Sidereal Time along as 17h 38m 13s this area also shows the 10th house as 25° Sagittarius (for this type of reference you need to know the symbols); when we go to the 5th row down we see the heading latitude. Being that Los Angeles latitude is 34° we follow the left hand column down to 34 and follow it across to the closest sidereal time as above, referring to the top of the column it shows 11 which refers to 11thhouse, then 12, 1, 2, 3 each being house cusps.   When we run our figure down that 11th house is 17.7 to convert the figure after the decimal point we multiply the .7 by 6 which converts it to 42'. Here the result is 7° 42'. This is the simplest way of figuring out 7/10 of 1° or 60'. In the Table of Houses the sign Capricorn appears under the 11th house and so the 11th house cusp will be 7° 42' Capricorn.

Converting 12th House

In looking up the cusp of the 12th house in the Table of Houses we find 14.4. .4 is again multiplied by 6 giving us 24' therefore 12th cusp is Aquarius 14° 24'. The Aquarian symbol is found under the cusp of the '12' house at the top of the column.

The 1st House

The first house is *never corrected*. It is copied exactly *as it appears*. In this case we find Pisces 21° 38' as found in the Table of Houses.

The 2nd House

The cusp in the second house is given as 2.4. The 4 is again multiplied by 6 for a result of Taurus 2° 24'. If you cast your eye up the column of the 2nd house you will note there has been a sign change from Aries to Taurus. This can occur in other columns so you must always check.

The 3rd House

The cusp of the 3rd house is given as 1.5. The 5 is multiplied by 6 gives Gemini 1° 30', notice again the sign change that occurs in the column.

The remaining 6 houses cusps are placed under opposing signs using the same degrees and minutes that have been calculated. For example 25° Sagittarius is on the 10th house, the house which opposes that is the 4th it's cusp will be 25° Gemini. 11th house cusp is 7° 42' Capricorn the opposing cusp will be the 5th house where the cusp will be 7° 42' Cancer.

PROPORTIONAL LOGARITHMS

	Hours and Degrees												
	0	1	2	3	4	5	6	7	8	9	10	11	

The tabular data in this proportional logarithms table is too faded and low-resolution to read reliably.

Using the Proportional Logarithms

If we go back to the beginning and now look to the 6th step we find we have 10hrs 24min with adding the True Local Mean Time and the Equivalent Greenwich Mean Time. With this information we can use above Logarithms.

Finding the 10hr column and then the 24min row we see the junction shows .3632 with this we now apply it to the individual planets movement.

We need to work out the difference between each of the planets on the 7th to the 8th. This calculation is below

Sun on 7th was 15° Scorpio 11'
on 8th   =16° Sc 11'   exactly 60' = 1°
                     The total movement for 24hrs.

The following is the calculation for finding all planets movements
Sun 15° Sc 11'. First each 1° contains 60 minutes so we deduct 11 from 60.

$$
\begin{array}{r}
60 \text{ min} \\
11 - \\
\hline
= \quad 49'
\end{array}
$$

$$
16°\text{ Sc }11' \quad
\begin{array}{r}
+11 \\
\hline
=60 \text{ min} \quad = 1°
\end{array}
$$

Going back to the Logarithms we see 1° is 0' is 1.3802 we then add the Constant Logarithm .3632

$$
\begin{array}{l}
1.3802 \\
+.3632 \\
\hline
1.7434
\end{array}
$$
we go back to the logarithms which shows 0hrs 26m

Sun position on 7th
$$
\begin{array}{r}
15°\text{ Sc }11' \\
+\;0°\quad 26' \\
\hline
=15°\text{ Sc }37'
\end{array}
$$
Sun position for 10hr 24m

The next example is the Moon this has the fastest calculation as it moves around the Earth not the Sun and the least distance from the Earth. Going by the ephemeris the moon is 0° Sagittarius 50' on the 7th November. It had moved to 12° 39' in Sag the next day, now we calculate the exact difference between the 7th and 8th of November:-

Moon on 7th   0° Sag 50'
Moon on 8th   12° Sag 39   difference 11° 49

7th
$$
\begin{array}{r}
0°\text{ Sag }50' \\
+ \quad\quad 10' \\
\hline
1°\text{ Sag }00'
\end{array}
$$
  ⟶
$$
\begin{array}{r}
10' \\
+11 \quad 00'
\end{array}
$$

$$+ \quad 11 \text{ Sag } 00' \quad\longrightarrow\quad + \quad 39$$

	12	00
forwarded	12	00'
	+	39'

= 11 49 Total movement in 24hr

_8th Nov   12°   39'

In logarithms following the 11° column to 49th row we find .3077 (log. For ☽)
Now we add the Constant Logarithm to the difference between 7th and 8th Nov to find the adjustment of the moon.

$$\begin{array}{r} .3077 \\ + \quad .3632 \\ \hline .6709 \end{array}$$

Going back to the Logarithm we find .6709 is in the 5° column and 07 minute row. Moon 0° 50' Sag plus 5° 07'

+0 50' -= 5° Sag 57' Moon's position for 10hr 24

Venus position on 7th November was 9 deg Libra 10 min Venus is inside Earth's orbit as such will move faster than the Earth remembering the Earth moves around the Sun 1 deg every 24 hours, we therefore expect Venus to move further as shown below.

7th Nov   = 9° Lib 10'
8th Nov   = 10° Lib 22'   difference 1° 12'

7th   9° Lib 10'
$$+ \qquad 50' \longrightarrow \quad 50'$$
        10 Lib 00   +22
$$+ \quad 22 \longrightarrow \quad 72' = 1° 12'$$
8th   10 Lib 22

Log for Venus   =   1.3010
$$+ \quad .3632 \text{ (Constant Log)}$$
                           1.6642

        1.6642 reconverted through Logarithm is 32'
Venus on 7th   9° Lib 10'
$$+ \qquad 32$$
        9° Lib 42' Venus position for 10h 24m

Uranus position on 7th Nov `1972 it's the 7th planet from the Sun therefore with all outer planets with reference to the Earth will move slower, as the Earth moves 1 deg in 24 hours we would expect it to move very little, where the Earth takes a year to circle the Sun, Uranus takes 7 years roughly whereas Pluto takes between 12 and 32 years.

Uranus on 7th Nov '72 20° Lib 20'
                = Difference 4'
8th   20° Lib 24'

7th   20° Lib 20'

8th   +   04'
          20° Lib 24'   (4 minutes total movement in 24 hours)

Using the Constant Logarithm .3632 we add it to the log for Uranus

               2.5536 Log for Uranus
               + .3632 (C.L,)
               2.9195 this total reconverted 2'

Uranus on 7th = 20° Lib 20'
                +   02'
               20° Lib 22

90

Chapter 13 - Foods of Constellations etc.

In this section I have arranged foods as to Constellation, as each Constellation and it must be remembered that each Planet rules a Constellation and the food will apply to it. Along with Houses.

In creating a cure a combination found in plants can cut down the ingredients where you see the foods contain multiple ingredients; but, in fear of repeating myself, remember the opposite side & sign in a chart, if there are planets whether transiting, progressive or natal maybe affected negatively, and so there would be a degree of that planets /constellations and houses that plant would require. This is paramount where there is little orb from corresponding degree. Personally I've found the best formula is by using all the influences and a separate plant for the planet/constellation and house.

To combine it you need to look to the squares, oppositions, quincunx's aka quincunx's.

Example: Almonds contain two specific ingredients Magnesium and Silica these are under two separate planets Sun & Jupiter; If you go to 'The Anatomy' you will see which part of the body these planets rule.
* A clearer illustration of Chemical compositions can be found in Constellations & Their Chemical Composition

Foods of Constellations

Foods - Herbs / Vegetables & Fruit	♈	♉	♊	♋	♌	♍	♎	♏	♐	♑	♒	♓
A. Acacia			•							•		
Aconite												
Adder's Tongue												
Agrimony				•					•			
Almonds					•				•			
Aloes -	•		•			•			•			
Flowers											•	
Angelica					•							
Anise			•			•			•			
Aniseed			•			•			•			
Apple		•					•					
Apricot									•			
Archangel		•					•					
Artichoke		•					•					
Asparagus	•	•	•	•		•	•		•			
Avocado			•	•								
Avocado Peel								•○				
Azaleas			•									
B. Balm			•			•			•			
Banana				•								
Banksia										•		
Barley											•	
Barberry	•											

92

Herbs/Veg &n Fruits	♈	♉	♊	♋	♌	♍	♎	♏	♐	♑	♒	♓
Barren Wort										●		
Basil								● ○				
Bay Leaf					●							
Bay Tree					●							
Beach Tree										●		
Beans						●	●			●		
Beet (White)									●	●		
Beetroot									●	●		
Birch							●			●		
Birdsfoot												
Bitter Sweet			●									
Black Hellebore										●		
Blackberry		●					●					
Blackberry Spikes												
Blackthorn												
Bloodwort									●	●		
Borage							●		●			
Bramble							●					
Briony	●											
C. Cabbage				●								
Cacti	●							●	●			
Calendula					●							
Capers				●								
Capsicum	●			●							●	
Carraway			●									

93

Herbs/Veg &n Fruits	♈	♉	♊	♋	♌	♍	♎	♏	♐	♑	♒	♓
Carrot	●		●									
Cayenne Pepper	●											
Celery			●	●	●	●		● ○		●	●	●
Centuary -	●				●							
American												
Cherries - Winter		●	●									
Chestnut		●	●									
Chickpeas			●									
Chickweed				●								
Cinnamon			●				●		●			●
Cloves	●	●							●			
Cocaine - Coca											●	●
Coffee												●
Columbine						●						
Comfrey			●	●						●		
Coral-wort				●								
Cornflower				●								
Corn Hornwort					●							
Couch grass		●										
Cowslip		●					●					
Cranebill		●					●					
Cresses	●			●								
Croton Tiglium -											●	
G. Ginger	●											
Gooseberries		●	●									

Herbs, Veg & Fruit	♈	♉	♊	♋	♌	♍	♎	♏	♐	♑	♒	♓
Gourd				●								
Grapes		●		●	●							
H. Hare's Foot			●									
Hart's Tongue									●			
Heart Trefoil					●							
Hemlock										●		●
Hemp										●		
Holly										●		
Honeysuckle	●	●						● ○				
Hope	●											
Hops	●											
Horehound	●		●									
Horseradish	●			●								
Horse-Tongue	●		●									
House Leek				●					●			
Hyssop				●								
I. Iris				●								
Ivy							●			●		
J. Jasmine									●			●
K. Kidney Beans		●										
L. Laurel					●							
Lavender		●	●									
Leeks	●			●	●							
Lecithin	●			●	●							
Lemons -												

95

Herbs, Veg & Fruit	♈	♉	♊	♋	♌	♍	♎	♏	♐	♑	♒	♓
Wild lemons	●											
Lettuce				●					●			
Licorice												
Lily - of the Valley		●	●	●								
White			●		●							
Liverwort			●									
M. Madder	●	●										
Maidenhair			●									
Mandrake			●							●		
Mango				●	●							
Maple									●			
Marigold					●							
Marshmallows		●										
Mercury			●						●	●		●
Mint							●					
Moss												
Motherwort								●				
Mulberry			●				●					
Mushroom + Salt				●							●	
Salt												
Mustard	●								●			
Myrrh			●						●		●	
Myrtle (Wax)	●											
N. Nailwort			●									
Navelwort										●		

96

Herbs, Veg & Fruit	♈	♉	♊	♋	♌	♍	♎	♏	♐	♑	♒	♓
Nettle	●											
Nightshade								●				
Nutmeg									●			
O. Oaks									●			
Oats	●		●						●	●		
Oils * pain relief										●		
Olive					●				●			
Olive Spurger			●									
Onions	●		●							●		
Orange					●							●
Orris Root				●								
P. Parsley			●									
Parsnip			●									
Peanuts							●					
Pennyroyal							●					
Peony					●			●				
Peppermint	●				●				●			
Peppers	●											
W. Walnut					●							
Watercress	●											●
Whitlow Grass				●								
Wild Wallflower				●								
Willow				●								
Winter Greens				●								
Witch-hazel	●											

Herbs, Veg & Fruit	♈	♉	♊	♋	♌	♍	♎	♏	♐	♑	♒	♓
Wolf's bane										●		
Wormwood	●						●	●○		●	●	
Y. Yarrow												
Yew Tree												
Yacca												

ANIMAL MEAT & SEAFOOD	♈	♉	♊	♋	♌	♍	♎	♏	♐	♑	♒	♓
Ants -												
Fire	●							●				
Honeypot	●	●										
Beef -		●										
Brains		●	●									
Breast		●		●								
Heart		●			●							
Kidney		●					●					
Liver		●					●		●			
Mammary Gland		●		●								
Milk		●		●								
Neck		●										
Buffalo - Feral												
Water	●										●	●
Chicken -			●									
Anus			●					●				

ANIMAL MEAT & SEAFOOD	♈	♉	♊	♋	♌	♍	♎	♏	♐	♑	♒	♓
Breast			●	●								
Heart			●		●							
Livers			●						●			
Lungs			●									
Thighs			●						●			
Wings			●									
Banter eggs				●								
Crab				●								
Blue Claw Crab				●							●	
Blue Swimmer				●							●	
Mud Crab				●						●		
Red Crab				●								
Sand Crab				●		●		●				
Fish -	●										●	●
Mullet			●			●					●	●
Red Fish											●	●
Blue Fish											●	●
Silver Fish	●		●								●	●
Sword Fish												●
Shark	●							●				●
Goat -	●									●		
Ankles	●									●	●	
Brain			●							●		
Heart					●					●		

99

ANIMAL MEAT & SEAFOOD	♈	♉	♊	♋	♌	♍	♎	♏	♐	♑	♒	♓
Goat												
Breast			●	●								
Heart	♈		●		●							
Knees												
Livers			●						●			
Lungs			●							●		
Milk										●		
Thighs			●						●			
Wings			●									
Banter eggs				●								
Crab				●							●	
Blue Claw Crab				●							●	
Blue Swimmer				●								
Mud Crab				●						●		
Red Crab				●								
Sand Crab				●								
Fish -	●					●		●			●	●
Mullet			●			●					●	●
Red Fish											●	●
Blue Fish											●	●
Silver Fish	●		●								●	●
Sword Fish												●
Shark								●				●
Lobster - cooked		●										●
Octopus			●					●				
Oysters	●											
Rock Oysters											●	

◔ in the Scorpio column means the product needs to be Fermented. I felt the symbol of the ¼ Moon appropriate.

☞ Finger symbol in a column means there can be dangers to areas of the ruling planet and should be used sparingly

Where it involves meat and different parts this would work best with the Sun Sign of the individual e.g. Taurus person with a tumor in the brain may look to the brain of the cow/beef.

The grey areas are those foods I've used, and have been nearly all the meat and crustaceous foods except goat and other exotic foods that aren't found in the local supermarket. I've also trialled the Scorpion. Not good for hair when Scorpio's 8th house and Jupiter are in Aries which are opposed to Saturn, Jupiter rules hair and 8th house is ruled by Pluto/Scorpio everything or nothing Aries rules the head and Saturn shows blockages when opposite.

Some of the more interesting foods are from the Tables of Composition of Australian Aboriginal Foods by Janet Brad Miller, Keith W. James & Patricia M.A. Maggiore

The best foods I've found for cures have been those that are known as the Symbols given for each zodiac sign. E.g. Aries symbol is the Ram, the Ram is the male sheep, but, secondly the term is also used for a male goat, these two shouldn't be confused the Ram in astrology is that of Aries and the sheep family, the Ram in Capricorn is the Goat. As such, I often use sheep meat, lamb (common in supermarkets) for formulas; alternately Aries is a forger and rules sharp instruments it also rules items that appear sharp, this can be used in foods i.e. Wheat under Mars. These are alkaline as are all the uneven signs of the zodiac, but, as with many plants it can be altered this is seen with Tobacco it has a Mars and Neptune influence, which means it could give a neutral ph affect.

The next is the Taurus symbol which is the Bull, I have found beef meat has been successful in throat problems but mixed with oil; where it concerns a plant I look for sweet and earth plants, another animal that could be looked at is the snail, it eats vegetation and is slow as the bull in general, and so the snail can be used for throat problems and areas associated with Taurus and could also be ruled by Virgo as it's small. Their lactation is a substance that could be used in the pituitary gland or for excessive nose running, possibly just rubbed on the nose. I'm not suggesting you try it only that scientists could look into it, it is already an animal eaten by the French.

When doing formulas, a person needs to look at the planets affecting each other in particular the 150° angles, but this can also be found by planets that rules constellations that would otherwise be in 150° angle in a house that is making 150° angle. Therefore, you're looking for at least two types of foods.

GLOSSARY

(✷ This symbol the asterisk shows the aspects that are hardly used)

Ascendant - A degree and constellation calculated at the time of birth which is crossing the eastern hemisphere, illustrating the 1st house, it shows how you look and what your immediate environment would be like. And, is the where all other cusps are calculated.

* Bi-Quintile - a minor aspect needing more exploration, generally no longer used.

Conjuncts - Planets that are at the same degree or within a 8 degree orb for planets up to Saturn. Conjunctions are a focal point in the Birth Chart. Their effect is to lay positive or negative stress according to the Sign and House positions of the planets concerned.

Cusp - is the precise degree found from the Time of birth, and is organised by calculating the Ascendant. It may be confusing but each cusp occupies thirty degrees, important cusps are 1st, 4th, 7th and 10th, these are the active houses or non-submissive houses, that look at the immediate environment, home, long term partnerships and career path. It also pinpoints north, south, east and west degrees in a chart.

* Decile - a minor aspect needing more exploration, generally no longer used.

Geocentric Chart - places the Earth in the centre of the solar system.

Heliocentric Chart - places the Sun at the centre of the solar system.

Horoscope - a Greek term meaning 'hour watcher' a chart formed on the D.O.B. and time of birth is then created placing planets as seen in their constellations.

Intercepted signs - intercepted signs are more common in charts where the birthplace is found in more extreme north and south latitudes versus latitudes found near the equator. In the extreme latitudes a house will contain more than 30 degrees, and in this case we find an entire sign enclosed in it and therefore, without appearing on any actual cusp. Such a sign is called "intercepted". In the equal house system, intercepted signs in a chart cannot happen.

Meteorological Astrology - the application of the science to the forecasting of weather conditions, earthquakes and severe storms.

Midheaven - is the M.C. Medium Coeli it is the highest point in the sky taken from the Earths tilt at the time of birth

Mundane Astrology - is Astrology which is not based on understanding personalities which Horary is, it's based on the time something happens in the outer world i.e. a letter being received, a ship sinking, a volcano erupting etc.

North Node / South Node - These points are always opposite each other. They are mathematical points where the Moon's orbit intersects the plane of the ecliptic. Some say they are points of karmic like yin and yang. The North Node shows the areas that we need to develop, whilst the South Node are areas we need to develop less in, and have to learn not to fall back on. They are points that take into account the Sun, Moon and Earth at the time of birth.

Oppositions - accentuate the polarities in a Chart, and can also form a strong integrating link. A person needs to come to terms with the opposition by combining both.

Planets – The planets in astrology are those that stay within a 10-19 degree orb and are seen along the Sun's ecliptic/path, the same path that pinpoints the 12 constellations. The Sun is not actually a planet it is a Star, it is halfway thru its life cycle and is believed to have approx. 5 billion years left, but is considered a planet for convenience, in fact it is the opposite of Earth along, the Moon is also considered a planet which is in fact the Earths Satellite. As such there are 10 planets, 11 if we count the newly found Chiron Planet it is believed to be between Saturn and Uranus.

Progressions – One day 24 hrs from the birth time, equals one year of a person's life and equals the first year's progression, and, illustrates how the personality changes. It also indicates what the parents were doing and illustrates stages in their relationship.

Quincunx – is 150 degree angle with a 2-3 degree orb, it is said they are unpredictable but it's more likely that they are set off by transits or progressions. They can cause health problems.

* Quintile – minor aspect needing more exploration, generally no longer used.
*
Radix – a point of origin for a personal relationship.

* Semi-Docile – minor aspect needing more exploration, generally no longer used.

* Semi-Sextile – is a 30 degree angle, it is a minor aspect. This is a favourable aspect and enhances the meaning of whichever planets are involved. Semi Sextiles are the reverse to Semi-Squares they can make a person feel happy or optimistic but, not necessarily knowing why unless you look at the chart to see what planets are involved.

* Semi-Squares are weak aspects they can cause a person to feel annoyed but not sure why.

* Sesquiquadrate – is 135 degree aspect with 2 degree orb, it indicates strain and needs to be examined especially if found with more then 1 close planet.

* Sextile – is a 60 degree angle and makes an easy flow of air in a 360 degree circle, because of this angle it doesn't look into things deeply. Like Trines it can bring out the pleasant characteristics in a suitable subject. People can find it easy to work in the areas, which the planets show.

* Square – is a 90 degree angle depending on position, can indicate tension or give drive and strength to the character to overcome.

Solar Arc - Distance in degrees between the progressed Sun and the natal Sun. By adding this distance in degrees to the rest of the planets and points. Because the Sun moves at a rate of almost one degree a day, this method makes it rather easy to estimate positions of progressed planets and points. The degrees of progression are roughly equivalent to the age of the individual.

Square - is a 90 degree angle which can indicate tension, the person would have to try and bring these two aspects together to overcome the negatives and extremes.

Trine - A 120 degree an Angle, that shows favourable aspects. They are also helpful to a strong character but may exercise a spoiling effect on shallow people

Vertex - represents the intersection of the ecliptic and the prime vertical. It's considered an auxiliary Descendant. And found in the western hemisphere *as charts are on the reverse it would be found on the right hand side of a chart. As in the English language we read from the left. The Anti-Vertex is the point that is opposite the Vertex. Astrologers have found it important in relationships either meeting the significant other or the ending of that relationship. Some have found it also can indicate birth or death.

Often asked questions: -

Love - The question of true love and how to find it is often asked, below shows varying aspects that can cause a person to love whilst not necessarily being loved in return for the same reasons. Anything to last needs to be in a fixed sign.

Love is found when 1. A's Sun Sign is the same as B's Ascendant 2. When A's Sun Sign is on the Cusp of the 7th house in B's Chart. 3. If the girls Sun is in the same as his M.C. she will give encouragement and force to his aims. 4. Sun and Ascendant same sign. 5. Sun and Ascendant opposite gives considerable rapport. 6. Sun and Ascendant Trine or Sextile. 7. Aries and Scorpio quincunx but can be good. 8. Pisces and Leo quincunx, can be good. Usually quincunxes are not good.

Honour - is found when there are a number of planets in the 10th House

About the Author

As the author I wouldn't have felt compelled to write this book if I hadn't personally lived by what I've written. It's my hope that my research may help Astrologers become more involved in medical research. Everything has to begin with a basic formula which can be proved over and over again.

My compulsion for research first appeared when my family were very young where I began to look into personalities using Astrology to solve in-house fighting way back in the late 70's. In the 80's and 90's I ran a local newspaper, where without the co-operation of my family it would never have got out. Many a night we were walking around delivering it. The paper actually caused me to be involved in many local and rural areas and to look into the politics of our country with media releases from many branches of government. The volunteer programs, in neighbourhoods we covered, always needed prop up by the government who were always calling poor, whilst increasing their wages 3 fold.

Prior to closing the paper, I did a 2-year volunteer radio program researching every current affair program using astrology and its planets I realized how diverse the subject really was for even medical research on sudden curers were already defined as curers in astrology if they were only recognised this book is about recognising Astrology as a driving force for recognising those curers and delving deeper into complex curers.

When I saw my mother die in the early 90's having been turned away from Naturopaths where an operation was all too late. And seeing family members die before their time. I thought if we could read a person's personality using astrology why can't we look into medicine which history showed it was once used for.

I've put in a section under Foods ruled by Planets etc, in grey are the plants I've personally used. Of course I can't make the same formula for myself that I'd make for someone else and as I've got older and put myself in more confined spaces I've found it more difficult to do formulas for others let alone myself.

People want to know if there are quick curers, in some cases its hit and miss. You need to compare colours with foods and planets and get the final colour that would compliment both the disease symptoms and combined planet.

You need to know a bit about the anatomy for instance the Livers a blood red/brown. So a good food for people with Liver disease is to buy and eat liver or beetroot the same colour and preferably the same shape. I've tried to give all the elements that can be used e.g. minerals in cell salt, vegetables & herbs and where it can be found in animals, but why use an animal when we can use a vegetable or mineral.

I have diplomas and did a basic course in Astrology but I've been self-taught in the medical field mainly because there has been no one teaching medical astrology; But, I should add the extended studies have advanced through following the Runes, over many years, where I've been able to find the correlation; and, where I saw the correlation in the universe to the whole range of events good or bad which I was able to relate back in the terms of astrology and the many

Pisces traits I have.

I wish all those who try making formulas the very best don't forget you might need the runes as

well

The reason for my research, I guess you'd have to say is Death and what's caused me to write

this book is that whilst we have to accept death it shouldn't be premature

References

(If you haven't been to university you mightn't realise that the superscript numbering indicates the original authors or program as known at the time)

[1] Casenotes of a Medical Astrologer by Margaret Millard M.D.

[2] Encyclopaedia of Medical Astrology by H.L. Cornell, M.D. 1932

[3] The Australian Women's Weekly – Astrology Book by Richard Sterling

[4] The New Compleat Astrologer by Derek and Pauline Baker

[5] Collier's Encyclopaedia 1962 updated 1986

[6] The World Encyclopaedia 1971

[7] Solar Fire Astrology Software

[8] Chart our Own Horoscope by Ursula Lewis

[9] The Vitamin Bible by Earl Mindell

[10] Tables of Composition of Australian Aboriginal Foods by Janet Brad Miller, Keith W. James & Patricia M.A. Maggiore

www.ingramcontent.com/pod-product-compliance
Lightning Source LLC
Chambersburg PA
CBHW080021240326
41598CB00075B/696